St. John's Fever and Lock Hospital Limerick, 1780-1890

St. John's Fever and Lock Hospital Limerick, 1780-1890

By

Patricia M. Bennis

CAMBRIDGE SCHOLARS PUBLISHING

St. John's Fever and Lock Hospital Limerick, 1780-1890,
by Patricia M. Bennis

This book first published 2009

Cambridge Scholars Publishing

12 Back Chapman Street, Newcastle upon Tyne, NE6 2XX, UK

British Library Cataloguing in Publication Data
A catalogue record for this book is available from the British Library

ISBN (10): 1-4438-1393-1, ISBN (13): 978-1-4438-1393-8

TABLE OF CONTENTS

ACKNOWLEDGEMENTS

I would like to thank Dr. Chris O'Mahony, of the Limerick Regional Archive, Sr. Mary Morrisroe, former Matron of St. John's Hospital, and Fr. Mark Tierney of Glenstal Abbey, first for their kindness to me, and secondly for making available archival material.

I am indebted to Dr. Padraig Lenihan for his invaluable guidance and advice.

The library staff of the University of Limerick, Mary Immaculate College, Limerick City Library, The Regional Hospital Library, Limerick City Museum and members of Limerick Corporation all provided valuable assistance for which I am grateful.

The Maps of Limerick on pages 13 and 41 are Courtesy of the Leonard collection at the Glucksman Library, University of Limerick. John Ferrar The history of Limerick: ecclesiastical, civil and military : from the earliest records, to the year 1787 : illustrated by fifteen engravings, to which are added the charter of Limerick, and an essay on Castle Connell Spa, on water in general and cold bathing / by J. Ferrar. Limerick : A. Watson & Co, 1787. Rev. P. Fitzgerald and J.J. M'Gregor The history, topography, and antiquities, of the county and city of Limerick: with a preliminary view of the history, and antiquities of Ireland / By the Rev. P. Fitzgerald and J.J. M'Gregor, Dublin: Printed for G. M'Kern, Limerick, 1826-27.

Fig. 13 is taken from the Atlas of Irish History, Dublin 1997 edited by Seán Duffy, courtesy of Gill & Macmillan Ltd.

Lastly, a special word of thanks to my husband, Alan Bunworth, for his patience and support.

ABSTRACT

This study evaluates the role of St. John's Hospital in controlling the spread of fever, by admitting fever patients to hospital and isolating them from the rest of the community. In addition, large numbers of the sick poor received advice and medicine from the hospital, and doctors occasionally visited them in their homes. The success of St. John's in treating fever patients was based on a combination of routine hygienic practices which would have kept contagion to a minimum and aided recovery; the knowledge and ability of Dr. John Geary to distinguish different fevers; the nourishing food given to patients and the less-aggressive nature of their 'cures'[1].

This study deals to a large extent with the 1820s, and to a lesser extent with the 1840s a period when admissions to St. John's hospital peaked. The register of admissions, containing more than 10,000 patients, together with newspaper reports covering the period 1825-1826, provide statistical information to validate anecdotal evidence of this epidemic. The sustained improvement in treatment is evidenced by reductions in the ratio of deaths to admissions between 1822-1826.

When the Cholera epidemic of 1832 arrived in Limerick St. John's was fitted out in the belief that it would accommodate any number of cases that might arise. Though the epidemic was of short duration, 953 people died of Cholera in Limerick hospitals.

St. John's Hospital admitted more than 5,000 fever-ridden patients during the outbreak of famine fever in Limerick City in 1845, yet the average rate of mortality was 6.38 per cent. Admissions fell during 1846, but rose in 'black' 47. In spite of the moribund condition of some patients admitted with Cholera in 1849, a relatively low mortality rate of 7.75 per cent was maintained. Voluntary and ad hoc responses to epidemics worked in the various crises but were patently inadequate to cope with the volume of fevers in the Great Famine.

---

[1] Bloodletting was going out of fashion.

St. John's Fever and Lock Hospital Limerick

Before us die our brothers of starvation
Around are cries of famine and despair!
Where is hope for us, or comfort, or salvation -
Where - oh! where?
—Speranza[1]

[1] Speranza (Mrs. W.R. Wilde), 'The Voice of the Poor', in The Ballads of Ireland, Edward Hayes (ed.), Vol. 1 (Dublin 1855), p 349.

INTRODUCTION

In 1700, hospitals in Britain were few in number, employed few people, were financed mainly on a voluntary basis and treated a very restricted social group of patients for a limited range of complaints. Hospital doctors treated patients without payment out of a sense of philanthropic duty. The growth of towns and social mobility, the increase of middle class philanthropy and professionalization in medicine saw the hospital develop as an institution in the wake of economic and social changes. The enlightenment of the eighteenth century was the beginning of a process which transformed the medieval religious social-service system, but the rise of the hospital to a central position in medicine occurred after the French Revolution.[1] 'A radically new approach was taken to medicine, which placed the hospital at the centre of health care in Europe and North America.'[2]. The growth of public health corresponded with the rise of centralized government.[3]

The Utilitarian goal of achieving the greatest happiness of the greatest number was the driving force behind the reform of the social conditions of the poor, acting in accordance with the laws of political economy.[4] The legislator's function was to solve the problems of morals and provide the fruits of good government – subsistence, abundance, security and equality. This enlightened self-interest, the concept of the English political philosopher Jeremy Bentham, (1748-1832), saw the welfare of the poor and the indigent as a necessary obligation of Utilitarian government. When wages were unobtainable, relief of poverty became a duty of government which could not be left to private charity. He had an optimistic belief in the economic value of population growth as he planned for the relief of poverty. Restoring the sick poor to health, and hence, the labour market he saw as essential to the strength of the Mercantilist state (the idea that the strength of the state depended on its productive and trading wealth). Bentham's concept was a powerful force in the state provision of public health in nineteenth-century Britain.[5]

'General' hospitals were established in London and other British cities in the early-eighteenth-century. Their raison d'être was charity, to take in the 'deserving' poor such as labourers, who conscientiously tried to support their families by employment. Criminals, prostitutes and the destitute were considered to be largely responsible for their own plight and were regarded as 'undeserving'. Children, fever cases, and incurables were also excluded. The patient population consisted mostly of accident cases or minor medical problems. The middle and upper classes sought treatment at home. In the second half of the eighteenth century a number of new hospitals were set up - the lying-in hospitals for women in childbirth, lunatic asylums, smallpox hospitals and hospitals for venereal disease.[6]

At the end of the Napoleonic wars, Britain, free of the burden of military expenditure, increasingly directed more of the national budget to its domestic public health policy. A link was established between poverty and morbidity which underpinned the idea of State welfare. The costs to industry and society in general could be reduced by preventing premature mortality of breadwinners caused by epidemic disease. Gradually political measures were adopted to prevent epidemic disease created by rapid urbanization as the pace of industrialization increased.[7]

The Report of the Poor Law Commission in 1832 concluded that the system of public relief of poverty and destitution, provided by each parish, artificially depressed the price of labour and removed the incentive of the fear of hunger to the poor to help themselves. Edwin Chadwick one of the authors of the report believed that the answer 'was to deter pauperdom by making it less eligible than the lowest paid labour'[8] and this would be achieved by depriving the pauper of his liberty, split up his family and incarcerate them in a workhouse. The new Poor Law was set up under the Poor Law Amendment Act in 1834. Public health reform was widely criticized in the nineteenth-century by the Tory press, who claimed that any interference from the state into the lives of its citizens was gross paternalism which undermined the whole philosophy of individual freedom. Doctors, on the other hand, wanted greater powers of intervention for 'state medicine' put into practice. The Victorian state in Britain continued to expand and became increasingly interventionist.[9]

So to what extent is the history of St. John's hospital, founded in 1780 part of this wider pattern? St. John's hospital followed the trend set by hospitals founded in the early eighteenth century England which enlisted the support of a few aristocrats whose names were published prominently to encourage those of lower social standing to make donations. Friends, relatives and other contacts were also tapped for their support. Benefactors became hospital governors, who elected a dozen or so of their number to supervise the hospital.[10] However, there were also notable differences. St. John's was founded before the French revolution to care for fever patients, who, as we have seen, were excluded from general hospitals. The medical men employed there were paid a salary, nevertheless, their motivation would appear to be the Irish notion of Christian service to the community, as exemplified in the work of Doctors John and William Geary. The Hartstonges, who were of the ruling class, did not need the social status that might be gained by establishing a hospital, and so firmly was it established that it flourished after their deaths.

The Irish gentry didn't lack humanity, according to Ferrar, but they liked the good life. They grumbled about a small tax 'while Englishmen of the same fortune, and in a much dearer country, pay four shillings in the pound on their rents to support a Poor House in every parish'.[11] It was not until 1772 that the Irish House of Commons passed an Act, establishing Poor Houses and Work Houses in every county in the kingdom.[12]. Under this Act, in 1773 the County and City grand juries of Limerick presented five hundred pounds for the erection of the House of Industry, to care for, among others, the aged, the feeble poor, helpless infants and lunatics. "A gloomy abode of mingled want, disease, vice and malady, where lunatics were loaded with heavy chains and fallen women bound and logged", is one description of the house.[13] Over the years, as the number of inmates grew, the contributions dwindled. It was pitifully small and harsh but it was a beginning of care for the poor of Limerick.

The first hospital established in Limerick, in 1765, was located outside the City wall, in St. Francis's Abbey on ground given in perpetuity at a peppercorn a year by Edmond Sexton Pery.[14] Fifteen years later St. John's Hospital was founded, in 1780, by his sister, Lady Harstonge, a kind and intelligent woman who, from her visits to comfort the sick poor in their miserable homes, saw the need for an institution which would care for fever patients in a large and populous district. By isolating the fever patient the risk of contagion to other family members was reduced. Cures could be effected through reducing the temperature by bathing, and building up the strength of the patient with nourishing food. Before 1780 there was no provision for the hospital treatment of fever patients "St. John's being the first building of the kind erected in the empire".[15] They suffered and died in their homes under the combined pressure of poverty and disease. In the eighteenth century the word 'fever' usually encompassed typhoid, typhus and *purpura* (both confusingly called 'spotted fever'), and relapsing fever, and epidemics were frequent.

Smouldering cases of fever were always to be found in the poorer districts of towns. Fever originated among the lower classes, but was not always confined to them.[16] Trying to make sense of epidemics Barker and

Cheyne, two Dublin physicians, who wrote a contemporary account of the recent fever epidemic, (in 1821) said:

> That certain classes of disease arise suddenly among a people previously healthy, and having increased for a series of months or years, then gradually decline or altogether disappear is well known to every observer. The causes which render sickness at certain times thus epidemical, are also in some instances sufficiently obvious. .... But why fever, which is at all times present in countries where many or most of the inhabitants must be susceptible of its attacks, should at particular times become epidemical, does not so easily admit of explanation.[17]

Before the discovery of microbial pathogens late in the nineteenth century, the prime source of disease was believed to be 'miasma'; - poisonous gases given off by unhealthy environments such as stagnant water, body odours and rotting animals and vegetable matter. Dr. Bernard Kavanagh, writing in 1863 on the sanitary state of Limerick, quotes Doctor W.J. Cox, an eminent writer on sanitary science:

> animal and vegetable emanations are a fruitful source of zymotic disease; that these noxious agents operate as causes in regard to the whole class of epidemics; that what will, in one place, develop the exciting cause of typhus, will, in another, produce scarlatina, smallpox, or cholera: and that the baneful gases which constitute the pablum of zymotic poison, are constantly being generated in places abounding in filth.

Dr Geary, senior physician in St. John's hospital, likewise, accepted that contagion spreads disease; he also observed on numerous occasions, new outbreaks which he could ultimately trace to the poor. Believing that overcrowding and filth caused disease, he claimed that it began through the 'concentrated putrid air'. The dwellings of the poor were a source of 'concentration of the putrid effluvia', produced as a result of keeping pigs, grains, beer, and a heap of fermenting potato skins in a small room, 'adding to the impurity of the air'.[18] Walking through the parishes of the old town, or even some of the leading streets of St. Michael's parish, he encountered in each 'a quantity of concentrated putrid matter, sufficient to impregnate the circumambient air with contagious effluvia, and thus, in an already enfeebled and wretched population, engender and propagate infectious disease'.[19] An outside agent was not always thought necessary as noxious vapours, by reaction, produced fever in the very body they arose from. Dr. Geary believed that famine was an important pre-disposing factor rather than a 'cause' of fever. In medical terms, we now know that the 'cause' of typhoid, typhus, dysentery, smallpox, etc., was quite different in each case but, doubtless, malnourishment was a major predisposing factor.

Excluding epidemic fevers, tuberculosis was usually the major cause of death in the seventeenth and eighteenth centuries.[20] An ancient disease of humans, it flourished in the crowded and filthy cities of Europe and Asia.[21] It accounted for as many as one- third of all deaths; Bills of Mortality show that 427 out of 2,193 Protestant deaths in Dublin, in 1743 were due to consumption.[22] No figures are available for Catholics, or for Limerick city, but it is probable that they were similarly affected. The colloquial names for tuberculosis, as given in the 1851 Census Report were 'decline', 'decay' (of youth or manhood), pulmonary consumption, hectic fever, neglected cold, abscess of lung, tubercular consumption, as well as phthisis or consumption.[23] Since none of these terms are mentioned in St. Johns Fever Hospital report, can one infer that there were no tubercular patients admitted? Irish folklore suggests that consumptives were kept at home, since people did not know the cause of the infection, or how it was spread.[24] There was also a natural desire of the families affected to conceal the disease, according to Deeny.[25] Tuberculosis caused long-term welfare and economic problems and was normally considered a death sentence. Fever was a symptom of Tuberculosis; other symptoms included night sweats, coughs and difficult breathing, blood-spitting, and loss of weight. Diagnosis was difficult as all symptoms might not be present and none were peculiar to tuberculosis. Continued ill-health was, perhaps, the best indicator of the presence of the disease. It progressed in unpredictable ways. Cases which appeared to be advanced might recover spontaneously while young adults often died very quickly, and for this reason the disease came to be known in the nineteenth century as 'galloping consumption'. Though it was essentially a young adults disease, it was also found in infants and children – though most died from infantile convulsions, pneumonia, diarrhoea and enteritis. Tuberculosis affects all parts of the body, but pulmonary tuberculosis, in which the lungs are diseased, was most common. Children were more likely to suffer from tuberculosis of the bones and joints which led to crippling, or to tuberculous meningitis which was invariably fatal.[26] The lymph nodes of children were sometimes affected by the disease (formerly known as scrofula), which deformed the features and Lupus which ate away at the face. Alternatively, it could attack the abdomen, the central nervous system, or the skin. Consumption was a disease of the poor who were under-nourished and lived in overcrowded, insanitary conditions. Ingesting infected milk or meat caused the disease and coughing and sneezing spread the infection.

Voluntary hospitals in the nineteenth century generally excluded incurable diseases such as tuberculosis, according to Lynda Bryder, because doctors wanted to show results in terms of cure.[27] This, however, will not explain why the disease is not recorded in the archives of St. John's Hospital, since it was a Fever and Lock Hospital, and there was no cure for venereal disease at that time. Venereal diseased patients very often remained in the hospital for months, and one patient with a sore leg was kept in the hospital for 313 days. Dr. Geary, writing of the reluctance of the sick to go to hospital in the early days says "the poor of this country are more warmly and affectionately attached to their relatives than those of almost any other", they preferred to keep the sick members of the family at home and give them personal attention despite contagion.[28]

Contagious disease is that which can be transferred to another person by ordinary social contact, in the home or workplace. All contagious diseases such as measles are infectious, but many infectious diseases, such as typhoid or syphilis, are not contagious (being transmitted by food or water which is contaminated by infected human excreta, or by sexual contact).[29]

The hospital began in a guard house of the citadel of St. John and with just a few beds attempted to prevent the spread of fever by removing patients from their dwellings. In spite of limited funds a decision was taken in 1785 to demolish the guard-house, and erect a new purpose-built hospital. During the rebuilding in the year 1786, the patients were transferred temporarily to a house in the Englishtown by the Abbey River, near Harstonge's town house, not far from Baal's Bridge. The present hospital opened for the reception of patients in July 1787. From the outset, large numbers of the sick poor received advice and medicine from St. John's hospital "and were occasionally visited by the medical officers in their houses, a practice which continued 'till January, 1797, when a Dispensary was established". Geary notes from the records that the externs treated were 13.25 to 1 intern or 32,453 to 2,591.[30]

Established primarily as a fever hospital, one ward was set aside for the treatment of women suffering from venereal disease. More commonly called Sexually Transmitted Diseases today, infections are contracted primarily, but not exclusively, by sexual intercourse. Until very recently they were thought to be limited to syphilis, gonorrhoea, chancroid and lymphogranuloma venereum. The latter two are found mainly in tropical countries but St. John's patients included sailors, soldiers and other travellers,[31] so it is possible that these infections were treated under the generic name of venereal. Herpes is the only named venereal infection.

Syphilis and gonorrhoea were thought to be manifestations of the same infection until 1838 when it was established that they were in fact different diseases.[32] A mother infected with gonorrhoea could transmit the disease to her baby during childbirth. The acquired infection, gonococcal opthalmia, is a severe inflammation affecting one, or both eyes, but the commonest cause of blindness in children was opthalmia neonatorum, a non-venereal condition.[33] Children could also contract gonorrhoea by sharing a bed with infected parents.

Syphilis is interesting from a medical and historical point of view. This infectious disease can simulate many diseases in the fields of medicine and surgery; and can be transmitted to children. It has a long incubation period which caused difficulty in diagnosis as a venereal disease, and when the symptoms manifested themselves it was not realized that they were the result of an infection acquired many years previously. It has three stages - primary, secondary and tertiary. Mercury was used to cure syphilis in the sixteenth and seventeenth centuries. Dr. William Wallace of Jervis Street Hospital, introduced potassium iodide to treat the disease in 1835.[34]

Congenital syphilis is an infection acquired during fetal life, from the mother. Unless treatment is given to a pregnant woman in the primary or secondary stage of syphilis, there is little chance that the infant will be born normal and healthy, but ‘this is the disease of exceptions and all kinds of variations are both possible and likely’. Infants who are severely affected by early congenital syphilis have a rash, bone abnormalities, jaundice, enlargement of the liver and spleen, and are very prone to infections such as pneumonia or gastroenteritis. Among other abnormalities which may appear later are deafness, inflammation of the cornea, and peg-shaped teeth.

When Columbus went to America in the fifteenth century members of his crews mixed freely with the local Indian inhabitants, who are believed to be the source of a new infection. By 1521 when Fracastorius wrote his famous poem ‘Syphilis Sive Morbus Gallicus’ and gave the disease its name, it had been spread all over Europe by soldiers and mercenaries returning from America. It was carried by Portuguese sailors to India and the Far East. Syphilis was first recorded as a major epidemic in Europe at the end of the fifteenth century. It raged among the French army. The soldiers returned to their homes, and the disease quickly became known as the ‘French disease’. It was for a time extraordinarily virulent, became milder over time and by the eighteenth century it assumed the form we know today.[35]

Whenever epidemics of fever or dysentery broke out venereally diseased patients were discharged from St. John's Hospital in order to provide more accommodation for fever patients. The only other Lock hospital in 1841 was in Dublin. Established for females affected with venereal diseases, they were total outcasts from society, and remained and died in the Lock and other hospitals. Because of the moral guilt attached to this disease the census returns would not be accurate and male deaths may have been returned as dying from other causes, such as diarrhoea or dysentery, both of which are frequent symptoms of the latter stages of this disease. Wilde observed a decrease in virulence and fatality in venereal disease between 1820-40.[36]

Lady Harstonge was the wife of Sir Henry Hartstonge, who was one of the two Limerick County MPs in the Irish Parliament.[37] To secure permanent revenue for a growing hospital, Sir Henry introduced a bill, which was passed in 1781, making an annual grant of £100.

The hospital was managed by a board of subscribing Governors who appointed from the board a committee of management. In 1850 there were 19 life Governors who originally paid £21 each and 7 annual Governors. While the board was predominantly Protestant ascendancy in composition, the staff, including the hospital doctors, were mainly Catholic. The first Doctor appointed to the hospital in 1780 was Dr. Hassett. He was succeeded by Dr. Crump who contracted typhus fever from one of his patients and died in 1796. Then Dr. Grogan came in 1796 and attended the sick of the hospital until June, 1818. With the increased admissions, convalescent wards were established at his suggestion, to give relief from noise and intrusion and frequency of relapse. To cope with the epidemic of 1801, Dr. John Geary M.D. was appointed as its second physician. The visiting apothecary, Mr. H. W. Baylee, became resident in the hospital and was a member of the Management Committee and treasurer to the hospital. The staff at first consisted of a housekeeper, nursetenders who cared for the fever patients and the victims of venereal disease, and a porter.

Notes

[1] Lindsay Granshaw, 'The rise of the modern hospital in Britain' in Andrew Wear (ed.), Medicine in Society, Historical Essays (Cambridge 1993). pp 197-199. (hereafter Granshaw, Medicine in Society).

[2] Ibid.

[3] Dorothy Porter, Health, Civilization and the State, A history of public health from ancient to modern times. (London 1998) pp 49-50. (hereafter Porter, Health, Civilization and the State).

[4] Ibid. p 116.

[5] Ibid. pp 58-61.

[6] Granshaw, Medicine in Society, pp 201-205.

[7] Porter, Health, Civilization and the State pp 109-111.

[8] Ibid. p 117.

[9] Ibid. pp 77-78, 112

[10] Granshaw, Medicine in Society p 201

[11] John Ferrar, The History of Limerick, (Limerick 1787). p 225. (hereafter Ferrar, The History of Limerick).

[12] Ibid. p 223.

[13] Paddy Lysaght, 'The House of Industry', The Old Limerick Journal No. 4, September 1980, p 21.

[14] J. F. Devane, MD, A History of St. John's Hospital Limerick, (Limerick 1970).p 24.

[15] John Geary, M.D., A Historical and Medical Report of the Limerick Fever and Lock Hospitals, (Limerick 1820). Pp 9-11. (hereafter Geary, A Historical and Medical Report).

[16] F. Barker and J. Cheyne An account of the rise, progress and decline of the fever lately epidemical in Ireland together with communications from physicians in the provinces and various official documents Vol. I (Dublin 1821) p 418. (hereafter Barker and Cheyne An account of the fever lately epidemical).

[17] Ibid. p 24

[18] Geary, A Historical and Medical Report p 30.

[19] Geary, A Historical and Medical Report p 24.

[20] James Deeny, MD, Tuberculosis in Ireland - Report of the National Tuberculosis Survey (1950-53) (n.p. 1954). P 14. (hereafter Deeny, Tuberculosis in Ireland).

[21] K. F. Kiple, 'The History of Disease' in Roy Porter, (ed.), Cambridge Illustrated History Medicine, (Cambridge, 1996) p 37. (hereafter Porter, Cambridge Illustrated History of Medicine).

[22] Deeny, Tuberculosis in Ireland p 14.

[23] Deeny, Tuberculosis in Ireland p 11

[24] Deeny, Tuberculosis in Ireland p 12.

[25] Ibid.

[26] Lynda Bryder, Below the Magic Mountain, a social history of tuberculosis in twentieth century Britain. (Oxford 1988), p 5 (hereafter Bryder, Below the Magic Mountain).
[27] Ibid. pp 22-23.
[28] Geary, A Historical and Medical Report p 23
[29] Dr. Tony Smith, (ed.), Complete Family Health Encyclopedia, (London 1992), p 301. (hereafter Smith, Complete Family Health Encyclopedia).
[30] Geary, A Historical and Medical Report p 15.
[31] Ferrar, The History of Limerick p 137 The Swallow Packet, bound for Madras, sailed on February 21, 1781 from the port of Limerick.
[32] Ambrose King and Claude Nicol, Venereal Disease, (hereafter King and Nicol, Venereal Disease).
[33] King and Nicol, Venereal Disease pp 214, 215.
[34] J.B. Lyons, Thrust Syphilis Down to Hell and other Rejoyceana, (Dublin 1988) pp 36-37. (hereafter Lyons, Thrust Syphilis Down to Hell).
[35] Smith, Complete Family Health Encyclopedia, pp 255, 490, 532, 904, 966. Lyons, Thrust Syphilis Down to Hell, pp 22-23. King and Nicol, Venereal Disease, pp 1, 2, 3, 99, 100.
[36] W. R. Wilde, Esq. Reports of the Commissioners appointed to take the Census of Ireland for the year 1841, p xxiv,
[37] Prior to the Act of Union.

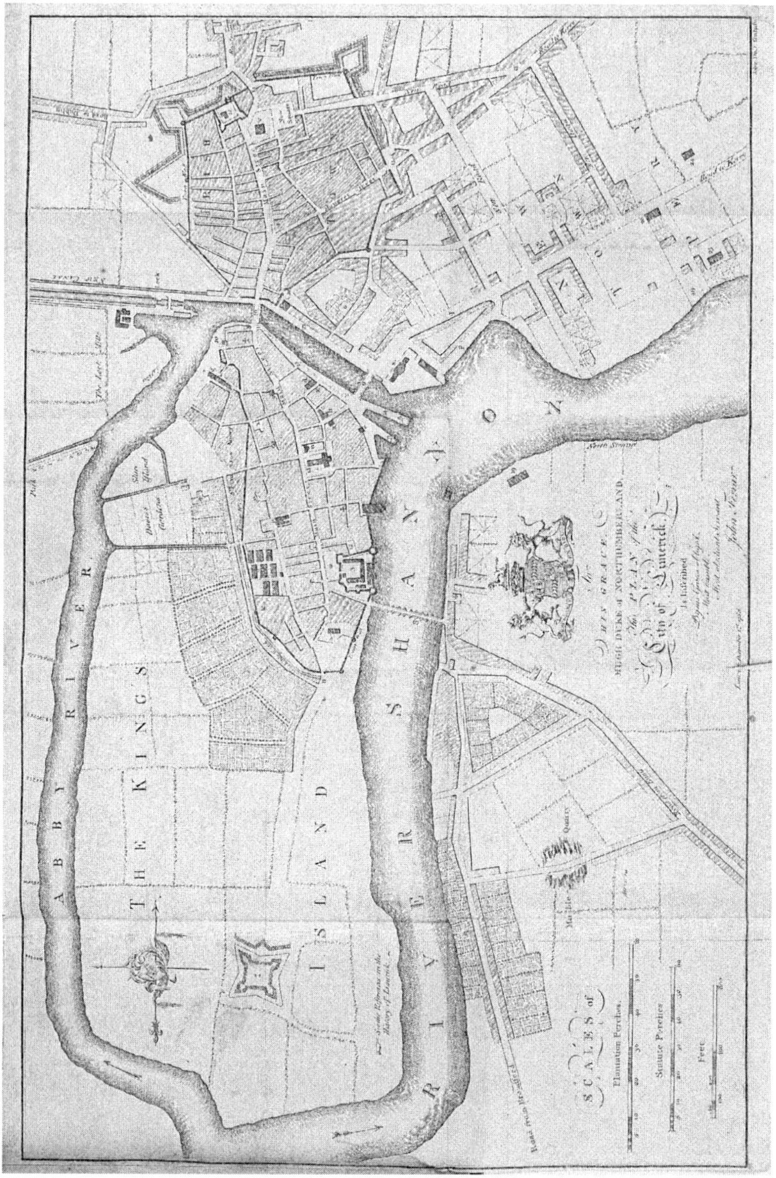

Plan of the city of Limerick 1787 Ferrar.

CHAPTER ONE

POVERTY AND PUBLIC HEALTH - LIMERICK 1750 - 1800

From the Treaty of Limerick to the insurrection of 1798 Ireland enjoyed a period of relative internal peace, troubled only by local, though sometimes serious, agrarian disorder.[1] After the siege of Limerick, the inhabitants, who numbered about 11,000,[2] reconstructed their houses and for sixty years a strict discipline was observed in the garrison. Strong walls and seventeen gates, which were locked nightly and every Sunday, encompassed the medieval city, preventing a free circulation of air through its narrow alleys.[3] The city consisted of two towns joined by Baal's Bridge, which spanned the Abbey River. The Englishtown on King's Island, with 218 houses, covered an area about twice the size of the Irishtown, which had 111 houses, predominantly stone built or 'cagework' (timber-framed houses filled with wattle and daub) structures, interspersed with thatched cabins.[4] One street, with each section known by a different name, ran the entire length of the city from St. John's Hospital to King John's Castle. They were John Street and Broad Lane (now Broad Street), Baal's Bridge and Mary Street. The oldest part of the city was the Englishtown (a c.1589 map shows the walled circuit of the Irishtown enclosing many gardens and orchards) and the newest Newtown Pery. In general, the older parts of the city had the most decrepit housing, decaying into densely packed warrens of the swarming poor.

Between 1731 and 1773 Philip Roche, one of the richest merchants in Munster, built a great many warehouses which transformed the Mardike (now Maradyke), and the slobland surrounding it, into Maradyke and Assembly, (now part of Charlotte's Quay), and Custom House and Arthur's Quays.[5] He also built houses on Patrick Street and Rutland Street, while Patrick Arthur, built a uniform row of houses along Arthur's Quay. A new bridge linking the Englishtown to the quays was constructed in 1761, and was replaced by Mathew Bridge in 1846. The city wall between Baal's Bridge and Quay Lane now Bridge Street was removed, creating George's Quay, and in 1764 the quay was extended to the canal. A plan for raising the new city of Newtown Pery, at South Prior's Land, was formed and the population of Limerick started to grow more rapidly from this point on.

The following graph[6] may, in fact, have significantly underestimated the city's population. A well-informed contemporary like Geary could plausibly maintain that the population of the city was 100,000 in 1820; more than three times the census figure! What matters here is not the absolute figure but the trends suggested by the data of rapid increase, tapering off somewhat by the 1820s and 1830s.

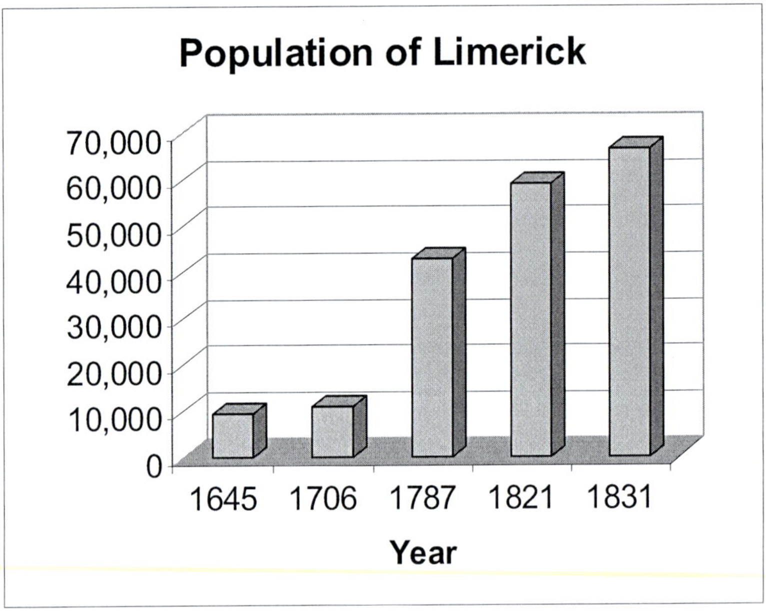

Fig. 1

The leases granted by Pery reveal that the area by the river was first developed, followed by the turnpike road leading south from Mungret gate. The overall Newtown Pery development was completed around 1830. The new town would in the course of a few years replace the old. It was advantageous to trade outside the city walls where the corporation could not levy taxes, but it was detrimental to the medieval city and led ultimately to its decay. This decay was compounded by high tolls which, apparently, deterred many producers from selling corn in the city; Mr. Richard Parsons, a local landlord writing in 1761, complained of the "Corporation vampires"

> in short, they have made me tired of farming, for I can assure you on oath, that these twenty years back except the last two years, that I sent into Limerick upwards of five hundred barrels of corn, but I was so oppressed with the usage I got in Limerick that I would not be any longer in their power, and have entirely quit tillage, nor have I sent one barrel of corn into Limerick those two years past, or ever will till the times alter.[7]

The Mayor, Sir Christopher Knight, in 1786, tried to improve the older city. It was paved and lighted with globe lamps. The ancient projecting windows, pent houses and signs were taken down, and streets named and signs fixed at street corners.

The relative peace and stability provided conditions for the growth of commerce and it flourished by 1740, trading with England, Holland, France, Spain, and the West Indies. The meat trade was enormous. Cattle were bought at Ballinasloe Fair, slaughtered in Limerick and the meat salted. It was then exported, supplying naval contracts and the West Indies. Other exports in 1776 included pork, butter exported in casks, hides and rape-seed. With such a trade in meat there must have been a good deal of offal available to the lower classes. The price of food items noted by Young (in 1776-78) are as follows; trout and eels sold at 2d. a pound and salmon at 1 1/2d.; wheat, 1s. 1d. a stone; barley and oats, 5 3/4d. to 6d. a stone. A 20 tons boat load of turf, cost 45s. A labourer would earn about 8d. per day. Even the moderately well-off could afford servants and keep a carriage and there were seventy privately owned carriages in Limerick by 1770. There was work for two coach-builders and a coach spring maker, for several victuallers and of course many labourers to load and off-load ship's cargo. Males and females, in great numbers, were employed in J.N. Russell's linen factory on the North Strand.

During the latter part of the eighteenth century, for want of other quantitative information, the health of the army may serve as an indication of the health of the community at large.[8] Limerick was the headquarters of the south-western military district, and had four army barracks - the Castle barracks in the Englishtown, the New barrack beyond Newtown-Pery, the Artillery barrack, in the Irishtown, and an Infantry barrack, in St. John's Square. Between them they could quarter 64 officers, 1,285 infantry and cavalry, and 158 horses. The hospitals could accommodate 124 patients and a military prison, in the new barrack, has 6 cells[9]. Until the commencement of the Crimean War in 1853 the garrison consisted of three regiments of infantry.[10] Exact numbers are not available as the strength of each company varied considerably. By keeping strengths low the government could maintain the maximum number of battalions at the lowest cost. In time of war, it was simpler to expand existing battalions than to create them from scratch.[11] Several regiments were stationed in Limerick where the markets were well supplied, and provisions cheaper than in other Irish cities.[12] In 1757, for the first time since the siege, English regiments enlisted Catholic soldiers in Limerick.[13] Three years later, Limerick was declared to be no longer a fortress and work on dismantling its walls and other defenses began.[14] The pace of expansion outside the medieval boundary quickened. The troops were generally in billets or temporary barracks, and consequently mixed more with the poorer classes from whom they contracted fevers and venereal diseases. English and Scots soldiers frequently suffered greatly from fever or dysentery, during the greater part of their first year's residence in Ireland.[15] Married soldiers lived out of barracks with their families, in the poorer parts of town, prey to whatever disease stalked the lanes and alleys of Limerick.

On 27 of December 1739 an intense frost accompanied by a piercing East wind set in and continued with little interruption for forty days. It was followed by unparalleled miseries. The Great Frost played havoc with the potato crop, and the ripened potatoes left in the fields were rendered inedible as a direct result of being frozen.[16] Food was so scarce that the following summer wheat sold for just over 2 shillings a stone or more than double the normal price. While food prices doubled other prices plummeted. Land and wool prices tumbled, while a boat load of best turf could be had for 14s. 1740 saw the onset of famine, which continued into 1741 when fever, which had been frequent, became epidemical and raged throughout the country. 400,000 people are reported to have died of famine and disease in Ireland[17]. The mortality was greatest in Munster where the poor were even less-well provisioned than elsewhere. St. Mary's cathedral Parish in Limerick recorded burial levels at this period greater than four times the 1737-39 average, peaking between February and July 1741[18]. In Limerick:

> A man might walk from John's gate to Thomond bridge without meeting six persons then. When the victims of cold and its attendant starvation became so numerous, that coffins could not be provided in sufficient quantities or with sufficient quickness, a bottomless coffin was provided,

> from which the corpse was thrown into the grave, and hundreds of the dead were interred in this way.[19]

According to Lenihan, the poor ate anything that would sustain them, including cats, dogs, mice, carrion, putrid meat, and nettles, and when they died of starvation their bodies lay unburied in the public streets. By the beginning of 1741, the accumulation of months of bad food, malnourishment and insanitary living conditions produced a number of epidemic diseases. John Rutty, an English-born Quaker doctor, identified four - smallpox, 'bloody Flux' (dysentery), malignant or spotted fever (i.e. typhus), and intermittent fever (relapsing fever) - each with a distinctive pattern or symptoms.[20] The first was an outbreak of smallpox following the long drought of the spring of 1740, when a surge in vagrancy accelerated the spread of the infection. Death by smallpox, was sometimes double, sometimes even triple that of fever in Dublin in 1740.[21] Smallpox, a highly infectious viral disease, transmitted from person to person was characterized by an illness resembling influenza and a rash that spread over the body and eventually developed into pus-filled blisters. The blisters became crusted and would sometimes leave deeply pitted scars. Complications included blindness, pneumonia and kidney damage. There was no effective treatment for the disease which killed up to 40 per cent of its victims.[22]

In the south of Ireland, Dysentery, 'the bloody flux', (so-called because of the frequent passage of bloody stools) was the primary scourge, first among the poor, then among other classes. The disease is caused by the dysentery bacillus and the infection is spread by flies, attracted by the stagnant pools for making dung-pits beside their doors, and by contaminated food or water. The disease would last from a few days to a fortnight, bringing with it extreme nausea, aching limbs, fever, colic, extremely painful intestinal ulceration and possibly internal gangrene, and bloody diarrhoea.

'Continuous' fever appeared in the final months of 1740; this may have been typhoid fever, and there were outbreaks of relapsing fever. The principal killer fever of 1741 was typhus. Both typhus and relapsing fever are caused by the infected faeces of human body lice, which breed in the squalid and over-crowded conditions of the cold and hungry poor. The typhus infection can enter the body through scratches on the skin or by inhalation, while relapsing fever is generally contracted through the skin. Typhus symptoms include under-skin haemorrhages and a prominent rash, high temperatures, bloodshot eyes and delirium. The immediate cause of death was usually heart failure. High temperature, generalised aches and pains, nausea, vomiting, nose bleeding and jaundice are features of relapsing fever. The fever ends after five or six days with a sharp crisis attended by profuse sweating and exhaustion. The symptoms return after about a week and there may be several such relapses before the disease runs its course. The official response to the crisis was to advocate public works which could employ all that would work, (since charity encouraged idleness), and clear the country of vagrants. This was a cruel response to the enormous food shortage, as most of those in need were too sick and debilitated to work. From the poor the fever spread to the rich and the Mayor of Limerick, Joseph Roche, Esq., was one of its victims.[23] The first attack was usually mild and thought to be merely a common cold, with a slightly faster pulse rate during the first six or seven days. As the disease advanced most of the patients exhibited petechia; and later still delirium or even frenzy, followed by coma. Symptomatic sweats produced no relief in this fever.

The ulcerated sore throat - which came to be known as Diphtheria, was very malignant and fatal to children in 1743, particularly in the countryside.[24] Diphtheria is an acute bacterial illness that causes a sore throat, fever, and sometimes more serious or even fatal complications. It was a major cause of childhood death worldwide until the first half of last century. It was necessary to cut the windpipe and insert a tube through which the child could breathe until the terrible infection passed, though even then the child frequently died.[25]

There was a marked increase of fever which began in the summer of 1771 and peaked towards the end of 1772. It resembled continued fever except that it was accompanied by a tremor of the whole body, incessant delirium, clammy and foetid sweats, and the petechiae were almost black.[26] That this was associated with privation is suggested by the fact that a riot broke out in Limerick on May 12, 1772, when a famished crowd attacked the lock mill looking for bread. The Mayor, Mr. Christopher Carr, called out soldiers who shot dead three rioters. The following day, rioting brought the 24th regiment into the main street of the Irishtown where three more people were killed.[27]

During 1786-87 and again 1791-92, a deadly 'putrid fever', as it was called, was widespread in Limerick, among all classes of society. According to Geary, this was typhoid, and was endemic in the city.[28] The first symptom is usually severe headache, followed by fever, loss of appetite, malaise, abdominal tenderness, constipation, and often delirium. If treatment were delayed, severe or even fatal, complications developed. Typhoid is infectious but not contagious, being spread by contamination of food or water by infected human excreta. In areas of poor sanitation, flies carry the bacteria from infected faeces to food.[29] In September 1761, a pump was erected at the head of Peter's Street, at the expense of Edmond Sexton Pery. He also cut a channel, nearly two miles in length, to bring water from Drumbanny into the Irishtown. This proved inadequate and another pump was erected near St. John's church in 1773. Ferrer in 1787 claimed that "these pumps are of the utmost service in cleansing the city,"[30] and indeed they must have supplied water for drinking and washing also. Flood water if it gets into the domestic supply can contaminate it. The river Shannon on reaching Limerick divides at King's Island, and the more rapid, narrow stream called the Abbey River regularly flooded Sir Harry's Mall in the old town. Flooding was also a problem in Newtown Pery where the houses were built with basements that extended under the pavements, giving access to sewers. Before pipes were fitted to convey waste from the houses it was carried down by the servants in sanitation buckets and emptied into the sewer. A heavy shower of rain would cause water to rush through the sewers and clear them. Although fifty miles from the Atlantic, the Shannon is tidal in this region and the back-flow in the sewers caused by high tide or the swollen rivers due to excessive rain, flooded these basements.[31] An outbreak of Typhoid could be caused by symptomless typhoid carriers handling food, such as domestic servants. Carriers are those who after recovering from typhoid fever, continue to harbour typhoid bacteria in the gallbladder, and shed them in the faeces for many years.[32] It is also possible that the pumps themselves were contaminated.[33]

While economic conditions were broadly favourable in the latter part of the century, in April 1791 high food-prices and starvation resulted in a mob breaking into a sloop loaded with meal, at a Limerick quay, and removing it. They later looted food from a warehouse in the town.[34]

From 1794 to 1798 fever, with a few exceptions, was of a mild type according to Geary.[35] Prolonged rain during the summer and autumn of 1797 prevented the peasantry from saving turf.[36]

Troop movements increased during the long-threatened rebellion of '98. From 1793 the formation of the militia and the recruitment of Catholics to its ranks, meant that the army was drawn from the native (though not local) population. Early in 1798 fever and dysentery increased considerably in the south and west and affected the troops. However the summer was so benign that the regiments on service often slept in the open air with no ill effects. According to Geary, the rising brought famine and fever in its wake; even in Limerick which saw little military action.

In the latter end of 1798 fever began to spread among the inhabitants and the troops. The regiments affected, included the Coldstream guards, stationed at Limerick. Fever was sometimes complicated with pneumonia or dysentery and the proportion of deaths to recoveries was so great that the Physician General, was requested to ascertain the nature of the fever and suggest the best means of dealing with it. The health of the army improved and in July 1799 all regiments were healthy, but continuous rain, and very cold weather caused the crops to fail. In the month of April 1800 a malignant fever appeared in a majority of the regiments of the Dublin garrison. The army in the south of Ireland was similarly affected; for example, of 2,620 soldiers stationed in the Cork region 123 died in a 16 week period. The conditions of the poor in the principal towns in Ireland in the years 1799-1802 were miserable. Waterford established a fever hospital in 1799 for the accommodation of the destitute. For their daily subsistence, the poor pawned their clothes, which increased filth, exposed them to cold, and crowding several members of a family into the same bed. Smallpox and dysentery accompanied this outbreak.[37]

Contagious fever continued to rage in the autumn and winter of 1800. The sufferings of the poor, and of the early cases of fever in the upper classes, Dr. Osborne in Cork observed, caused benevolent people in some cities, including Dublin, Cork and Kilkenny to set up Fever Hospitals to meet the emergency. The summer of 1800 was unusually dry and hot, and for several weeks the day-time temperature seldom fell below 70 degrees. Autumn was cold and wet and the crops failed again. Corn was imported and the distillation of spirits from grain was prohibited. The price of bread and potatoes, both of bad quality, together with other essentials rose to new heights.[38]

The following table, commencing 24th June, 1794, shows a substantial increase of admissions into St. John's hospital in 1799-1800, - almost double that of any year since its foundation.[39]

	Admitted	Cured	Died	Average mortality
1794-5	29	25	4	1 in 7
1795-6	49	44	5	1 in 10
1796-7	58	54	4	1 in 14
1797-8	61	54	2	1 in 30
1798-9	52	49	3	1 in 17
1799-1800	100	59	6	1 in 16
1800-1801	320	268	17	1 in 19
1801-2	411	413	21	1 in 19
1802-3	86	89	9	1 in 8

Fig.2

In 1800 and 1801, the Fever epidemic assumed 'an alarming aspect', according to Dr. John Geary, who was appointed to the staff of the hospital at this time. The apothecary became resident in the hospital, in order to help the two physicians at their work. The numbers affected were so great that it was impossible to accommodate all who sought admission. To remedy this, huts were erected by the friends of the sick, on roadsides and at the sides of fields throughout the country, where many must have died of famine and disease. Dr. Geary himself suffered for 21 days from Typhus gravior.[40] He recovered, and served the hospital for another twenty years. In February 1801, the Director General of Military Hospitals reported to Government:

> that the disorder with which the troops have of late been affected has been communicated by contagion, and that a fever of a dangerous and frequently fatal kind very generally prevails throughout every part of Ireland, which is ascribable to a deficiency in the usual quantity of food, a calamity which has for some time been heavily felt by the poor.[41]

In Dublin, wealthier classes were discouraged from buying potatoes, the staple diet of the poor.[42] Bread was portioned out sparingly. Under the management of the Governors of the House of Industry, four kitchens were established by the charitable, at opposite quarters of the city, to supply the poor with soup at the rate of a halfpenny for a quart. This example was followed in the cities and towns all over Ireland, and also by many country gentlemen. The government response to the crisis was to finance large imports of rice and maize from America, which was distributed to the regions by the army.[43] However, an unusually abundant harvest later in

1801 alleviated the subsistence crisis though there was no immediate improvement in public health.

Dysentery began to appear in many parts of the country in September, due to the change of temperature and rainfall after the long hot summer. It was followed by scarlatina in November, and a malignant sore throat, prevailed among all classes and proved fatal, particularly among the poor. At this time also opthalmia was a very prevalent disease.

Dr. Geary in Limerick and a Cork doctor reported that typhoid was the predominant type of fever in 1801, and that it was less inflammatory. The fever in 1800 and 1801, generally ended on the 5th or 7th day by perspiration; but the disease was liable to recur. Though it affected the poor more than the better-off, it was much more fatal amongst the middling and upper classes.

In the spring of 1802 the epidemic was on the decline, and about the end of summer the improvement of the public health became still more evident.[44] St. John's hospital resumed its normal activity until the next big epidemic of 1817-1819.

Notes

[1] JC Beckett, A Short History of Ireland, (London 1971), p 104
[2] O'Connor Exploring Limerick's Past, an historical geography of urban development in county and city, (Newcastle West 1987) p.36 (hereafter O'Connor, Exploring Limerick's Past).
[3] Ferrar The History of Limerick p.83
[4] O'Connor Exploring Limerick's Past Pp 38-39
[5] Gerry Joyce, Limerick City Street Names, (Limerick 1995), p 10. O'Connor Exploring Limerick's Past p 43.
[6] This graph is based on Calhaldus Gilbin OFM 'The Processus Datarial and the appointment of Irish Bishops in the Seventeenth century', in Franciscan Fathers (eds) Father Luke Wadding (Dublin, 1957) p.573; Patrick J. O'Connor Exploring Limerick's Past p 36; John Ferrar, The History of Limerick, Pp.97-98; and the Census enumeration of 1821 and 1831.
[7] Maurice Lenihan, Limerick Its History and Antiquities, (Cork 1967) p 351 (hereafter Lenihan, Limerick Its History and Antiquities).
[8] Barker and Cheyne An account of the fever lately epidemical p.10
[9] Samuel Lewis, A History and Topography of Limerick City and County, (Cork 1980) p 123. (hereafter Lewis, History and Topography of Limerick).
[10] Ferrar The History of Limerick p.83
[11] Letter dated 22 July 1998 from Michael Ball, Head of the Department of Printed Books, The National Army Museum in Chelsea.
[12] Ferrar The History of Limerick p.83
[13] Ferrar The History of Limerick p.128
[14] Ferrar The History of Limerick p.83
[15] Barker and Cheyne An account of the fever lately epidemical p.12
[16] Barker and Cheyne An account of the fever lately epidemical pp 5-6
[17] Lenihan, Limerick Its History and Antiquities p.335. Barker and Cheyne believed that 80,000 was nearer the truth, Barker and Cheyne An account of the fever lately epidemical p.6.
[18] David Dickson, Arctic Ireland, (Belfast 1998), p 67. (hereafter Dickson, Arctic Ireland).
[19] Lenihan, Limerick Its History and Antiquities p.335.
[20] Dickson, Arctic Ireland pp 44-45
[21] Dickson, Arctic Ireland p 46. Barker and Cheyne An account of the fever lately epidemical p.7
[22] Smith, Complete Family Health Encyclopedia p 924
[23] Lenihan, Limerick Its History and Antiquities p.335, Dickson, Arctic Ireland p 43
[24] Barker and Cheyne An account of the fever lately epidemical p.7
[25] Smith, Complete Family Health Encyclopedia 360
[26] Barker and Cheyne An account of the fever lately epidemical p.8
[27] Lenihan, Limerick Its History and Antiquities p.360. Ferrar The History of Limerick p.132

[28] Geary, A Historical and Medical Report p 24
[29] Smith, Complete Family Health Encyclopedia p 1022
[30] Ferrar The History of Limerick p.129
[31] Judith Hill, The Building of Limerick, (Cork 1991). Pp 125-6
[32] Smith, Complete Family Health Encyclopedia p 1022
[33] John Snow Anaesthetist and Epidemiologist, 1813-58, By mapping the location of deaths from Cholera he pinpointed the source of the infection - the water pump in Broad Street in London in 1854. He had the handle removed and ended the epidemic. Cambridge Illustrated History of Medicine p. 376.
[34] Wyse Jackson, Robert, The Story of Limerick, (Cork 1973) p 65
[35] Geary, A Historical and Medical Report p 26.
[36] Barker and Cheyne An account of the fever lately epidemical P.11.
[37] Barker and Cheyne An account of the fever lately epidemical Pp.13-16
[38] Barker and Cheyne An account of the fever lately epidemical Pp.17, 435-6.
[39] Geary, A Historical and Medical Report p 85.
[40] Geary, A Historical and Medical Report.Pp.17-28.
[41] Barker and Cheyne An account of the fever lately epidemical p.17
[42] Ibid.
[43] Gerard O'Brien, State Intervention and the Medical Relief of the Irish Poor, 1787-1850, in Greta Jones and Elizabeth Malcolm, (eds.) Medicine, Disease and the State in Ireland, 1650-1940 Cork 1999. (hereafter O'Brien State Intervention and the Medical Relief).
[44] Barker and Cheyne An account of the fever lately epidemical Pp.17-20.

CHAPTER TWO

ORIGINS 1780 -1820

A great quantity of rain fell between July and October, the harvest season, of 1816. Corn remained uncut in October and November; and much of it was lost. Potatoes, which were the main food of the poor in most parts of the country, were small and wet, and probably not very nutritious. The scarcity was greatest about midsummer of 1817 causing extreme distress. In some districts seed potatoes were eaten; and blood drawn from cattle, and mixed with oatmeal, nourished starving families. In these years Dr Geary admitted patients into the hospital, who had not eaten a meal of any kind for days; others said that their chief sustenance came from boiled nettles and other esculent herbs. It was not uncommon for people to die suddenly from hunger.[1]

The sufferings of the poor were increased by the quality of the straw used for bedding which was often half decayed. Turf could not be cut and dried for use because of the wet weather, so clothes and bedding were damp. It was difficult if not impossible to cook food properly; or heat their homes or clean them; even personal hygiene must have been neglected for want of fuel.[2] To compound the problem, with the end of the Napoleonic wars and the transition to peace, agricultural depression led to mass unemployment in 1816 and 1817; the wartime demand for cereals (to make bread, a portable food, for large armies) dried up suddenly. Cereal production was labour-intensive, resulting in mass unemployment among rural labourers. Many tenants were unable to pay their rents. The price of a day's labour fell to sixpence, or even to fourpence, without food; and this at a time when potatoes, were selling at the rate of tenpence for the stone; a quantity insufficient for the support of a small family. In Limerick markets were reasonable but unaffordable due to lack of employment. [3]

The poor bore this hardship; rioting only when food shortage and unemployment were at their worst. For example, rioters attacked corn mills and stores in Limerick on the 6th of June 1817. Porters carrying bread, from bakers to their customers, were robbed of their cargo. The

Lord Lieutenant issued a proclamation recommending the wealthier classes to discontinue the use of oatmeal and potatoes in their families.[4]

Between 1816 and 1819 Typhus ravaged Ireland. This outbreak differed from the 'ordinary fever' which was ever present in the poorer districts of towns, in its frequency and severity. Limerick followed the general pattern of a sharp increase in 1817. The exception to this pattern was Cork where the disease peaked two years earlier, for some reason.[5]

Patients admitted to the fever hospitals in Dublin, Cork, Waterford, Limerick and Kilkenny 1805-1818

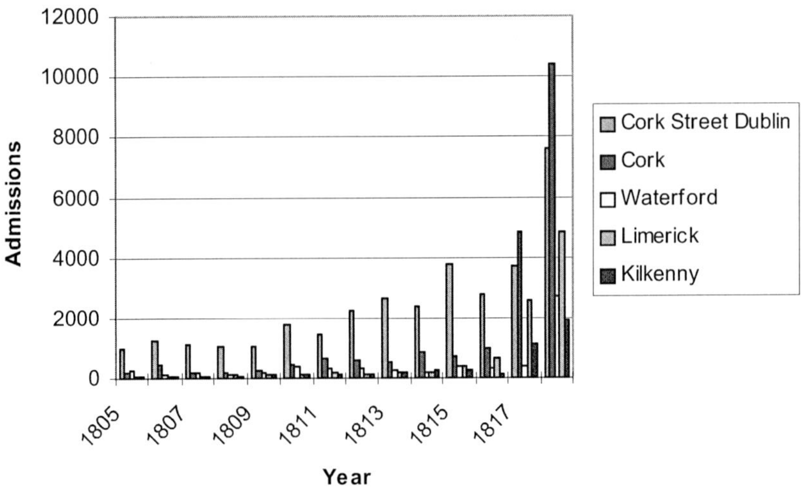

Fig. 3 Admissions to St. John's hospital were so great that to relieve the pressure a temporary hospital was set up nearby in The square on January 11th 1818. This hospital admitted 1,697 patients – 1,295 patients were admitted in 355 days. It closed on April 20th 1819. See Centrefold for this image in colour.

Females were more frequently attacked by Typhus than males, but it was more obstinate and malignant in males, probably due to their drinking habits; the blood being deprived of its oxygen by spirits and fermenting liquors, according to Darwin.[6] In the better-off orders of society the complaint was of shorter duration, more malignant, and consequently more fatal. One-tenth of the population of Limerick suffered from fever during the epidemic of 1816-19 and there were many cases of gangrene of the hips and shoulders. Terror and apprehension of the disease often creates a pre-disposition to it, according to Dr. Geary who cites a case where his nursetenders got alarmed and came down with mild fever for five or six days on admitting a woman with gangrene.[7] Gangrene of the feet was a common occurrence caused by prolonged wet, poverty, and exposure.[8]

Purpura differed from typhus in size and colour of the spots and in the way patients became suddenly anxious and depressed. The spots were large, mostly circular, and of a dark purple livid hue, and a few cases festered. Purpura fever, was almost indigenous to the Abbey in Limerick where, in some houses, three or four families occupied one small room. Adults suffered a considerable enlargement of the liver.[9]

Admissions to the Limerick Fever Hospital from 1803 to 1st December 1819

	Admitted	Cured	Died	Average
1803-4	95	85	4	1 in 24
1804-5	90	72	12	1 in 7
1805-6	86	88	3	1 in 27
1806-7	84	78	6	1 in 14
1807-8	110	91	13	1 in 8
1808-9	99	93	13	1 in 7
1809-10	105	102	4	1 in 26
1810-11	164	137	14	1 in 12
1811-12	145	145	12	1 in 12
1812-13	194	171	9	1 in 21
1813-14	200	196	7	1 in 28
1814-15	342	316	18	1 in 19
1815-16	381	350	22	1 in 16
1816-17	1275	1140	68	1 in 18
1817-18	2787	2381	226	1 in 12
1818-19	3153	2983	105	1 in 30
to Dec. 1st 1819	483	460	11	1 in 44
Total	9,793	8,888	547	1 in 17

Fig. 4

The increased mortality at Limerick was caused mainly by diarrhoea or dysentery, (rather than typhus) particularly in the autumn of 1818.[10] Dysentery was commonly associated with epidemic fever, and those who were already suffering from privation, damp and excess of whiskey were thought to be most at risk[11]. As the epidemic progressed, many relapsed, some several times.[12] Poor families shared one bed, often just a miserable wad of straw in confined and badly ventilated apartments[13]. In many instances, Dr. Geary says:

> I have seen the sick and well huddled together in the same bed without distinction of sex or age - the sick naturally confined in consequence of their illness, the well for want of clothes; which were consigned to a pawnbroker's shelf for days before, in order to sustain a miserable existence.[14]

A Cork doctor gives the situation a sharper focus:

> families, consisting of many individuals, were found in cellars and garrets, with no covering but the remnants of clothing too contemptible for even the pawn-broker's avarice, water their only drink, and food, if any, the offal collected from the slaughter-houses.[15]

The scene was the same in Palmerstown, in the back lanes of the Irishtown, in the Abbey and various other parts of Limerick, equally favourable to the propagation of fever.[16]

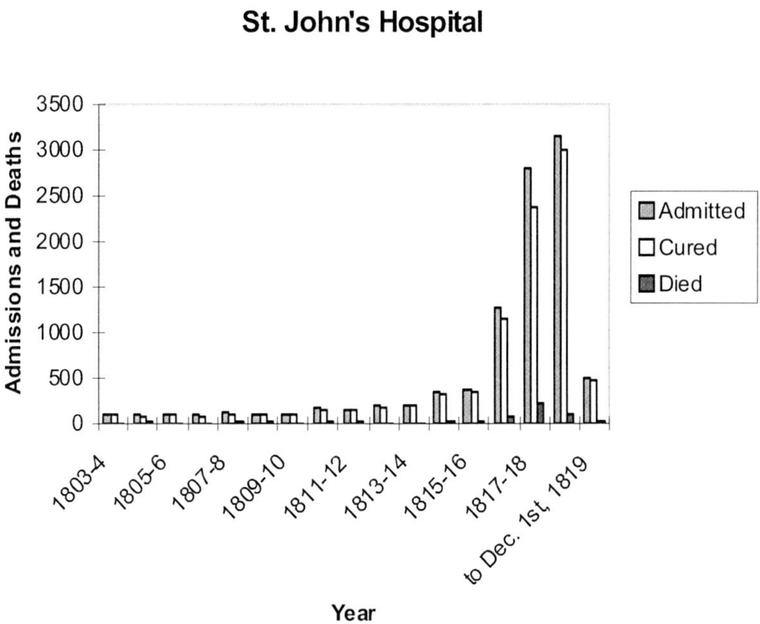

Fig. 5. See Centrefold for this image in colour.

The increased mortality in St. John's in 1817-18 was a result of the crowded state of the hospital that year. The numbers admitted were so great, (there were 243 in rooms originally designed for not more than 54 patients) that it was necessary to pass over tiers of beds to examine the sick. There were frequently forty people (four in a bed) in a room not exceeding sixteen feet square. Many died shortly after admission, of chronic dysentery and pulmonary infections, and less than a quarter died from fever. Mortality was highest in the twenty to thirty age group and only a small number of children died.[17] This epidemic was the largest that the hospital had yet experienced, and put an enormous strain on hospital resources. The committee appealed to the Lord Lieutenant to enlarge the accommodation at the hospital, but it was a local architect, Mr. Fitzgerald, who erected, at his own expense, a wooden building capable of holding 30 beds. The Government response was to legislate that Grand Juries were empowered to grant a sum of £500 yearly to Fever Hospitals.[18]

People with fever were removed to hospital, where it was the normal practice, immediately on admission, to cut their hair short, or even shave their heads. They were washed in vinegar and tepid water. Few patients came to the hospital before the third or fourth day, often too late to apply cold compresses and arrest the progress of fever. In St. John's, the bedclothes were changed once or twice daily. However, the patients returned home to the same infected beds and suffered relapses; sometimes fatally because they could not afford straw to renew beds, or fuel to heat water to wash bed clothes more frequently. With this neglect of cleanliness, fever spread through families. The practice of holding wakes was another source of contagion. Catholic priests attending the sick and dying suffered most. The lower classes were known for their hospitality even in times of want, and passing strangers were invited to share their accommodation. They were often rewarded by fever, even death.[19]

In Limerick, fever patients came from the same apartments, at intervals of one, two or three months. The disease continued for four years in a house near Mr. Kelly's tan-yard, in the lane leading to the Island, and for two years in a house occupied by Andersons in Fr. Davy's lane, Spittal, near Garryowen. The apartments of the patients removed to hospitals, were generally washed with quick-lime and water. It was believed that the use of nitrous fumigations and washing with lime diminished the frequent occurrence of fever in the same houses, but it proved more tenacious in others.[20] Church wardens were empowered by Act of Parliament to levy taxes within their parishes, to employ scavengers to remove noxious matter from streets and lanes and stop the spread of disease.[21]

As the epidemic fever drew to a close, there were still relapses. In many parts of Ireland mortality from smallpox was high. An epidemic catarrh appeared at the end of spring 1819, and in June and July, the ulcerated sore throat (dyphtheria) that was fatal to children, particularly in the countryside. The epidemic gradually burnt itself out and the hospital resumed its normal routine. In October scarlatina frequently occurred among children in parts of Munster.[22]

Having been a very old walled town, both the Irishtown and the Englishtown had many narrow filthy lanes, decaying houses inhabited from garret to cellar by a miserable population, including ejected tenants from the surrounding counties, in search of food and shelter for their starving families. Limerick because of its situation in relation to several counties attracted more than its fair share. The larger part of the Englishtown consists of the parish of St. Mary, with a history of destitution. St. Mary's was notorious for its extreme wretchedness, where the houses were in general more closely packed in, and there was, usually, a greater number of families to each house than in other parishes. Touching descriptions of individual suffering were given, by the Rev. Thomas Enraght, Catholic curate of this parish, and the force of those appeals brought contributions for their relief from various parts of England and even from India. The condition of the poor in St. Michael's and St. John's parishes was similar, wretched also, but not to the same extent as St. Mary's. The Parishes of St. Munchin and St. Patrick were mainly suburban and rural and were populated by the lower classes.[23] The New town was in the parish of St. Michael and in stark contrast to the old, consisted mainly of houses of wealthier shopkeepers, merchants and resident gentry of the city:

> Strangers, when they observe the elegance of the houses in this part of the town, the neatness of the equipages, and the gay dresses of the more respectable portion of the inhabitants, can never understand how Limerick can possibly contain so much poverty as is reported; and even the inhabitants themselves of this part, whose business scarcely ever leads them into the older portions, have little conception how human life is wasting within a few hundred paces of their doors. The medical men of the city, and the Roman Catholic clergy, could easily undeceive them.[24]

In 1824 a contract was made with the United London Gas Company to have the city lighted with gas. The original plan was limited to the New town but it was extended by the corporation to the Irishtown and Dublin Road, and by private subscriptions to part of the Englishtown.[25]

Dr. Geary, writing in 1820 estimated the population of Limerick at nearly 100,000.[26] In a report on the epidemic of 1817-19 the figure of 75,000 appears with a questionmark under population, when Dr. Geary noted that a quarter of the inhabitants suffered from fever in that epidemic.[27] The site of the city was not unhealthy. The population for the City of Limerick is given as 59,045 in the Census of 1821, with 36,447 in the City centre and 22,598 scattered over a large area of the suburbs and Liberties. This and the subsequent Census are regarded as greatly underestimated since the number of persons per house was rated at 11. This is not the image one gets from Thackeray or other visitors to the city of "a labyrinth of busy swarming poverty and squalid commerce as never was seen", where "every house almost was half a ruin and swarming with people".[28] The population increased rapidly between 1821 and 1851 in St. Michael's parish, which is mainly in Newtown Pery; and slowly in St. Mary's parish in the Englishtown, while it actually fell in St. John's parish, in the Irishtown, before the famine. The population of Ireland had increased enormously from 5 million in 1800 to about 7 million in 1821 in spite of the frequent pressure of great distress among the labouring classes of society and considerable emigration.[29] The population of the City of Limerick in 1831 was 67,575.

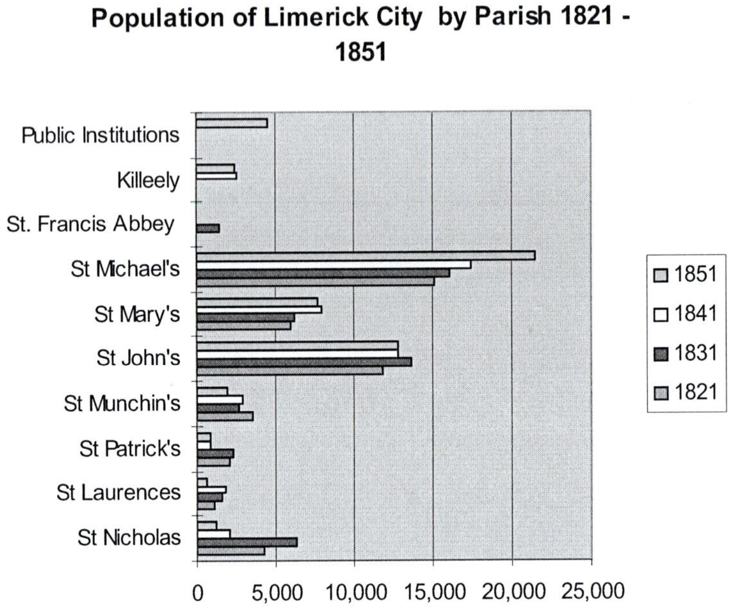

Fig. 6. See Centrefold for this image in colour.

No. of persons per house in 1831

St. Munchin's	St. John's	St. Mary's	St. Michael's
c.8	c.10	c.20	c.8

Clearly, St. Mary's was grossly congested, compared to other parishes and the number of admissions (per capita) to the Fever Hospital was more than one-third of parishioners. Admissions were increasingly from St. John's parish reflecting the growth between both census. St. Mary's Parish lost 37 houses in this period and gained a small increase in population. Dr. Griffin, a Limerick dispensary doctor, writing in 1841, of the mortality and fertility of the various city parishes notes that infant (under 3 years) mortality was highest in the inner city, reflecting the degree of poverty; St. Mary's at 55.28 per cent; in St. Michael's and St. John's the death rate was 51.87 per cent; and St. Munchin's parish was 45.61 per cent.[30]

The link between poverty and disease underpinned the idea of State Welfare, in European societies, but Malthus opposed State intervention and his influence was extensive. Writing in 1824, Malthus held that, unchecked, populations tend to grow at a rate that would double in size about every twenty-five years, while food supplies could not increase to the same extent. With preventive measures, such as self-restraint and delayed marriage individuals and nations could reap the rewards of better living conditions, but if these steps were not taken, then starvation, disease and war would keep the population in check.[31]

'Malthus blamed the endemic grinding poverty of the Irish, the famine of 1800-1 (which killed thousands of people), and even the political unrest of the 1790s, on overpopulation'.[32] The flaw in Malthus was his assumption that productive labour would, in fact, be available. Industry was in decline in some parts of Ireland from late 1810s and early 1820s and there was little industry in the city. The 1821 Census notes one industry in St. Patrick's Parish, a cotton factory which employed 52 people. In 1831 the returns give 23 males over 20 years of age employed in manufacture. Women's earnings were hardly worth counting, so that the whole family was mainly dependent on the man for support. If he became ill or disabled, then they very soon became destitute. Most adults on admission to hospital gave their occupation as labourer, they and their dependents made up the bulk of hospital patients. Labourers were employed about the stores and other places of business, when they could get work to do, which was difficult because of the failure of the 'industrial revolution' to take root. Artisans were slightly better-off but they too were bordering on destitution. Employment for women meant at any kind of drudgery that was available though they were capable of doing fine needlework. Those with entrepreneurial flair tried to carry on a little trade on whatever they could save from their husbands' earnings, in an effort to eke out a subsistence: "whole troops of pear-, apple-, and plum-women, selling very raw, green-looking fruit…".[33] It was also common practice to bring their best clothes to the pawn shop to raise a little cash on Monday morning and redeem the same item on Saturday evening.

> When the week's trade is unsuccessful, the coat remained in pawn, and on the Monday following some other article supplies its place; and so it goes on, until by some lucky chance they are again released, or, what is much more common, article follows article, until everything on which a penny can be raised is gone, and then comes the wind up. From this time forward there is a daily contest for even one day's existence, and the unhappy family is doomed to a course of privation and suffering.[34]

The opening of the Mont de Piété, a charitable pawn office, was intended to reduce the exorbitant interest charged on clothes pawned - in all about 735,956 items in a year.[35]

The source of the terrible living conditions was natural law, according to Malthus, and not as the utopians claimed, the result of social injustice. The solution, he claimed, was not public relief, which rather than diminishing the poverty and suffering of the masses would stimulate population growth and make the situation worse. The attitude to the poor was that their distress was caused by improvidence and vice; and that charity would encourage idleness. But Maltus was wrong, in a basic assumption that only suffering and the threat of still worse suffering could induce restraint in the masses. Abysmal poverty induces more of the same, and not prudence. The destitute survive by living just for the day. Only when incomes exceed the minimum is prudence possible.[36] Dr. Griffin, a dispensary doctor working with the destitute between 1822 and 1839, noted that 'production is often most rapid among a population in extreme wretchedness' and this he believed was due to the high mortality among infants and the aged.

> ….. as the poor nurse their own children, there is in general an interval of about two years between the birth of one child, and that of the next; but if a child dies early on the breast, this interval will be much shorter, and if this occurs often, there will be a certain number born as it were for the purpose of dying, and these being soon replaced, the same number may still be preserved as if there had been few or no deaths - or only the ordinary number.[37]

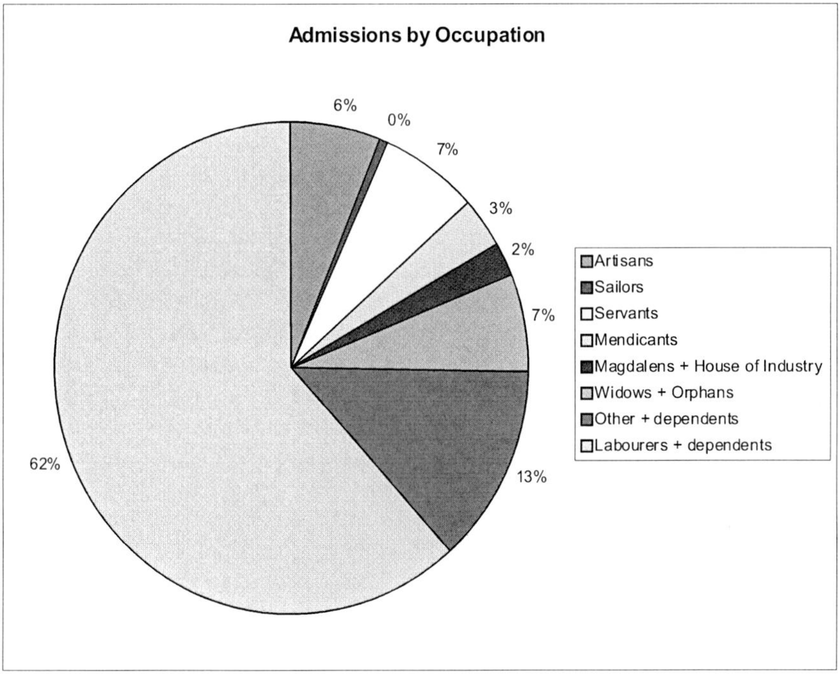

Fig. 7 St. John's Hospital Archive. See Centrefold for this image in colour.

There is no way of knowing how mendicants survived in the cities but the in the country they were better off than labourers; and fared best when prices were high:

> A beggar, by receiving a few potatoes at every house, will collect above four stone of them in the course of the day, which, at 4d. a stone, is 1s.4d., about double the sum which a labourer could earn in the same time: people were no less generous in a dear season. ….. during the scarcity of this year, it is said that the poor of the town [Askeaton] would not have known what to do, owing to the high price to which potatoes would have run, if it had not been for the quantities brought to the public scales for sale by the beggars!![38]

The Mendicity Association housed 200 'miserable objects' who would have to be turned out, adding to infection and disease of the city if sufficient funds were not raised.[39]

In England and Wales, the Old Poor Law 1795-1834 made each parish responsible for its own poor. A poor rate was levied on the inhabitants and work had to be provided for the able-bodied. A rising population following the end of the Napoleonic wars and agricultural depression created social and political unrest. Schemes for the reduction of expenditure on poor-relief included encouragement to emigrate for one million paupers and, according to Ó Gráda, was much more important than the trends in the birth-or death-rates.[40] Reform of the Poor Law Act in 1834 transferred the burden of relief to Boards of Guardians representing a 'union' of parishes, and elected by the ratepayers. No able-bodied man would receive assistance unless he entered a workhouse. Minimal medical attention was proposed. Doctors "tendered" for the care of a given district's paupers. A similar system was proposed for Ireland. Those who opposed it claimed it would put an impossible burden on the rates and merely aggravate the problem of Irish poverty or worse, they looked to the actual amount of destitution and sickness among the really poor, as a means of lessening the population. In 1838 the Irish Poor Law gave Ireland for the first time a system of poor law.[41] 'Limerick Union was the first to be declared (December 1838), and it had a new workhouse in operation by the middle of 1841'.[42] By the outbreak of Famine in 1845 there were 118 workhouses and each had its own infirmary. 'By 1846-47 the poorhouses had a capacity for over 100,000 inmates, but those qualifying for entry numbered around half a million.[43]

Notes

[1]Barker and Cheyne An account of the fever lately epidemical Pp.30-35. Geary, A Historical and Medical Report p.32

[2] Barker and Cheyne An account of the fever lately epidemical P.33.

[3] Barker and Cheyne An account of the fever lately epidemical. This is the wholesale price of potatoes. The retail price was of course greater. Pp.35-37. Geary A Historical and Medical Report Pp.35, 49.

[4] Barker and Cheyne An account of the fever lately epidemical Pp.40-41.

[5] Barker and Cheyne An account of the fever lately epidemical Pp434, 22. Geary A Historical and Medical Report P.31.

[6] Geary A Historical and Medical Report p.59

[7] Geary A Historical and Medical Report p.60

[8] Wilde. Report upon the Tables of Deaths to the Census Commissioners Census of Ireland for the year 1841 p.xxxvii. (hereafter Wilde. Report upon the Tables of Deaths).

[9] Geary A Historical and Medical Report Pp.50-51.

[10] Dr. Grogan in Barker and Cheyne. An account of the fever lately epidemical Pp.437-8.

[11] Geary A Historical and Medical Report p.77 Barker and Cheyne An account of the fever lately epidemical Pp.437-8.

[12] Barker and Cheyne An account of the fever lately epidemical P.439.

[13] Geary. A Historical and Medical Report p.47 Barker and Cheyne An account of the fever lately epidemical P.419

[14] Geary A Historical and Medical Report p.32.

[15] Barker and Cheyne An account of the fever lately epidemical 420.

[16] Geary A Historical and Medical Report P.33.

[17] Geary A Historical and Medical Report Pp.88-89.

[18] The Fever Hospital Act of 1818 and the Contagious Diseases Act of 1819 established The Board of Health. O'Brien Medicine, Disease and the State in Ireland, pp 200-201.

[19] Barker and Cheyne An account of the fever lately epidemical Pp.421-4. P.447. Geary A Historical and Medical Report Pp.47,49.72.75.

[20] Dr. Carroll August 1819 letter to Barker and Cheyne. An account of the fever lately epidemical Pp.447-8. Geary A Historical and Medical Report Pp.43-44.

[21] Geary A Historical and Medical Report p 83

[22] Barker and Cheyne An account of the fever lately epidemical Pp. 7, 448-9.

[23] Dr. Daniel Griffin, 'An Inquiry into the Mortality Occurring among the Poor of the City of Limerick', Journal of the Statistical Society of London, Vol.iii, part 4. (1841), p 306 (hereafter Griffin, An Inquiry into the Mortality)

[24] Griffin, An Inquiry into the Mortality P.307

[25] Lewis, History and Topography of Limerick, pp 122-3.

[26] Geary A Historical and Medical Report P.83.

[27] Barker and Cheyne An account of the fever lately epidemical P.83

[28] W.M. Thackeray, Irish Sketch Book, 1842, (Belfast 1985), p. 151.(hereafter Thackeray, Irish Sketch Book).
[29] Cormac Ó Gráda, Ireland A New Economic History 1780-1939 (Oxford, 1994). P.69. (hereafter Ó Gráda, Ireland A New Economic History)
[30] Griffin, An Inquiry into the Mortality Pp.321-22
[31] Introduction by Frank W. Notestein Three Essays on Population, (New York 1960) Pp.vii-viii. (hereafter Notestein, Three Essays)
[32] Ó Gráda Ireland A New Economic History p.4
[33] Thackeray Irish Sketch Book p.149.
[34] Griffin An Inquiry into the Mortality Pp.324-325.
[35] Mark Tierney, The Mont de Piété in The Old Limerick Journal No. 24 1988.
[36] Notestein Three Essays P.ix
[37] Griffin An Inquiry into the Mortality P. 320.
[38] Griffin An Inquiry into the Mortality P.327. P.328.
[39] The Limerick Chronicle 9 February 1825.
[40] Ó Gráda Ireland A New Economic History P. 74.
[41] Cambridge History of Medicine P. 317-20, Ó Gráda Ireland A New Economic History P.98.
[42] Chris O'Mahony, The Poor Law Comes to Limerick. The Old Limerick Journal No. 6 1980.
[43] Cathal Póirtéir, Famine Echoes, Dublin 1995, pp 115-117.

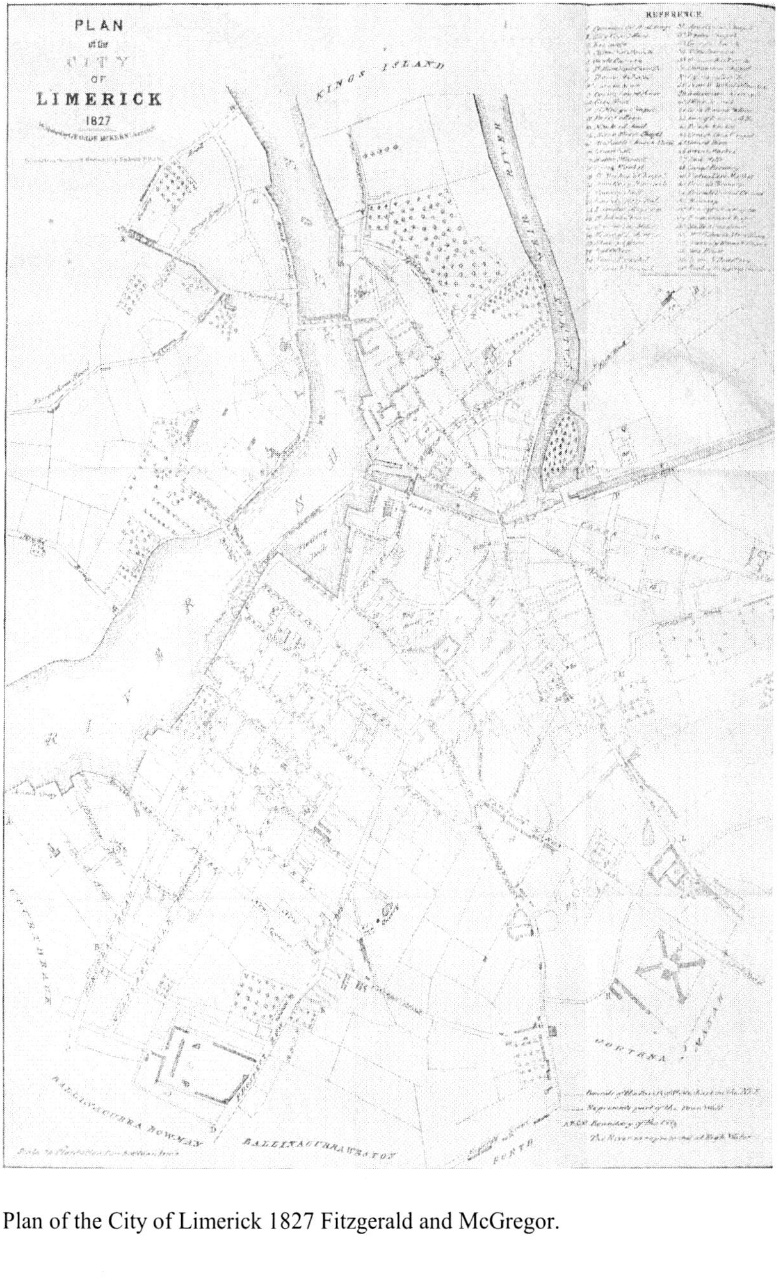

Plan of the City of Limerick 1827 Fitzgerald and McGregor.

CHAPTER THREE

1821 - 1826

The Register of patients at St. John's Hospital between 1821 and 1826 is incomplete. Four weeks records are missing as are particulars of the patients illness in several cases. Those admitted with fever numbered 8,360; 1,052 had venereal disease; 638 had dysentery; 11 smallpox; 2 measles; and 1 with whooping cough. In 1821, of 936 patients admitted, 247 had dysentery and more than half the deaths were from that disease. Mortality was highest in July, when 20 people died, but the disease proved fatal between August and December also. It was found necessary to discharge six venereally diseased patients after 5 or 6 days due to the increase of dysentery in the hospital. In 1822, ten per cent of those admitted with dysentery died,[1] but famine-induced diseases killed far fewer people that year, than earlier famines.[2] The number of patients admitted with dysentery was low after 1822, and it accounted for just one admission in 1826.

The following graphs (Fig. 8 and 9) show a marked increase in admissions in 1925-1826.

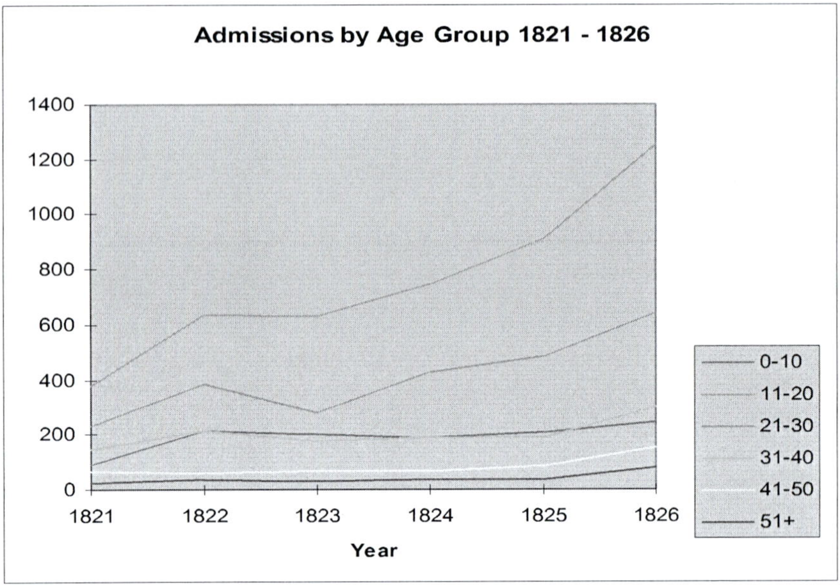

Fig. 8 St. John's Hospital Archive. See Centrefold for this image in colour.

People of all ages got fever but according to Dr. Geary, writing in 1820, it was more prevalent "when the animal spirits are most disposed to febrile excitability, that is from twenty to thirty, and from thirty to forty - next to those we find it most frequent in children under ten years"[3]. However, the register of patients admitted to St. John's Hospital covering the period 1821 to 1826 shows the most vulnerable ages to be those between 11 and 20 years old, - almost one half of all admissions were in this age group. The 21-30 age group comprised just a quarter of those admitted. One can only speculate why, in so short a period, this variable should apparently differ so greatly. The 1820s were economically depressed. Children from age 11 could make a contribution to the family budget, if only by maintaining themselves,[4] so of necessity they would need to be nursed to health as quickly as possible. Furthermore, there was a growing awareness of the excessive mortality among the children of the poor of the city of Limerick, - a rate much greater than that for England and Wales.[5] From a study of 1,017 families between 1822 and 1839, Dr. Griffin calculated the mean annual mortality to be about 5.05 per cent. While the deaths among the poor in this city were about 1 in 19 annually, among the well-heeled it was about 1 in 123 annually. He also noted, that 'the age of least mortality is also the age of least sickness, viz., 10 - 20'.[6]

Health care had improved the survival rate of all patients. Healing involves emotions and personal relationships between doctor and patient and all of the cultural factors which determine belief, identity, and status. In the nineteenth century, disease had to be liberated from the body. Physicians prescribed mild cathartics to aid the body in its efforts to expel the morbid material. Most diseases were self-limiting, their natural tendency even if untreated being to recovery not death. The good physician, cautious in his therapy, attempted simply to strengthen the body's vital powers in its struggle with disease. It was assumed that the symptoms of disease e.g. sweating, fever, or diarrhoea were modes through which the body sought to reestablish health. Little could be done for ills that were not self-limiting, so reliance was placed upon good food, hygienic conditions, and stimulants such as alcohol or relaxing anodynes such as opium. The physician's task was to understand the nature and timing of these healing mechanisms; to support, not undermine them. Physicians placed ever-increasing faith in the healing power of nature and the natural tendency toward recovery, moving away from remedies of purgatives, emetics and bleeding.[7] St. John's was fortunate in the quality of its medical staff. Hygienic practices in the hospital, which would have kept contagion to a minimum and aided recovery, included cutting patient's hair short or even shaving their heads, immediately on admission, and bathing and dressing them in clean bed clothes. Bed linen was changed at least once daily. Their diet was nourishing and included meat, bread and milk.

Ratio of deaths to admissions

1810-20	1820-30
1:13	1:20

Averages over decades conceal significant seasonality of admissions. The following graph (Fig. 9) reveals a fever 'season' from about May to September and peaking usually in July. The Poor Inquiry of 1835-6 established close connections between poverty, hunger and disease; when the potato was in short supply during the 'hunger months' of June, July, and August; the months when most admissions took place in St. John's Hospital.

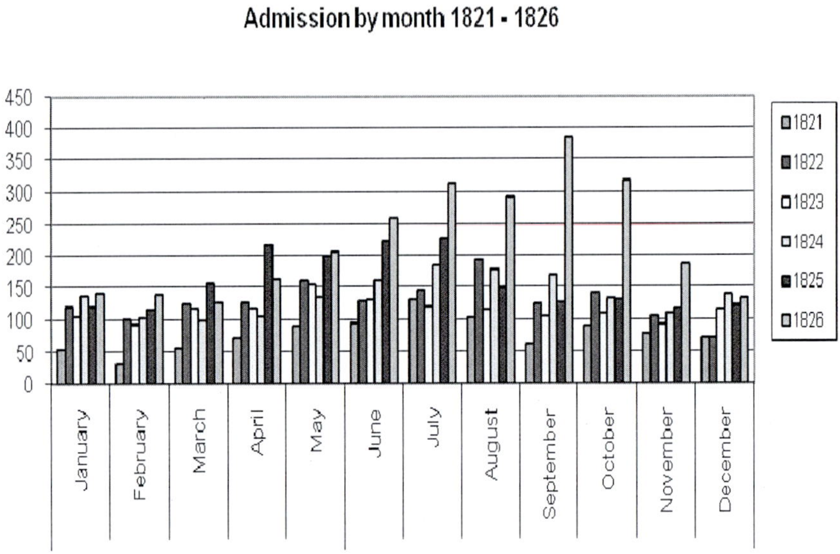

Fig. 9 St. John's Hospital Archive. See Centrefold for this image in colour.

> The distress of the peasantry is in proportion to the extent of time that thus intervenes, and the universal opinion that it is the most frightful evil in Ireland is but too strongly confirmed by the wretchedness that it annually renews or increase in the shape of regular periodic visitation which only varies from great privation to absolute famine, according the season, the price of food, employment and other local circumstances of the district.[8]

The pre-famine Irish had a high calorie diet due largely to the potato, which supplied good quality protein and different vitamins, supplemented with cabbage, turnips, and other vegetables. Nevertheless, they were still very unhealthy by today's standard. When times were hard the poor resorted to nettles, wild mustard, and other weeds. Only a very tiny fraction of Irish people starved in an average year and the poor could withstand a significant deficit in the harvest without undue excess mortality.[9]

The harvest failed again in 1822. Despite the increasing precautions taken against contagion, poverty increased the incidence of fever. The admission figures for St. John's hospital grew rapidly between 1821 and 1826 especially for fever patients but at this time, according to Wilde,[10] there was "no account of any pestilential Fever or other formidable epidemic occurring in Ireland, until the arrival of cholera in 1832-3." The hospital in its returns for the period 5 January to 12th April 1825 advised that 'fever has not prevailed to the same extent for the last 5 years'. Bedding could not be supplied because the funds were so low, and patients were obliged to share beds risking increased mortality. On 17th June shortage of accommodation was a problem for the increased number of patients, 76 having been admitted within a few days. On 16 July 1825 the attention of the public was drawn to the alarming increase of fever in this city and its vicinity, in the Limerick Chronicle. Contagion, among all classes of society, was contained to a degree by admissions to St. John's, but the applicants were so numerous that all the lock patients had to be discharged to create room for fever patients. Fifteen patients came in dying, ten of those in July. One patient died four hours after admission, while another lived for a further 31 days. A woman fever patient who was convalescent died suddenly of apoplexy. There were twelve relapse cases, one a sailor died after 6 days.[11]

The situation worsened in the following year. There were 468 inmates in the House of Industry in March 1826, which was unprecedented, and if they had the funds 56 'wretched room-keepers who had made application' would also have been admitted.[12] In St. John's, seven patients 'came in dying'. Relapse cases totalled 92 - in September alone there were 20 cases. The symptoms of the disease were not of the malignant type. The patients were affected with a low fever brought about by privation of food and clothing - some patients were absolutely starving. There were 1,746 admitted into the hospital within 9 months.[13]

On the 9th September a meeting of the inhabitants was called by the Mayor at the request of the Governors of the Hospital to discuss the alarming state of fever in various parts of the city, and the crowded state of the hospital. The Mayor invited his fellow citizens to address the meeting and Dr. Harding was first to speak. The fever cases had been so numerous, he said, that there was no alternative but to turn out all the venereal cases that had been in the lock hospital, to provide accommodation for the others.

> At present patients are lying on the floor between the beds; as the apartments are insufficient for their accommodation. The hospital wants funds to meet its increased expenditure and if something were not speedily effected by the inhabitants of Limerick the consequences to society would be most dangerous.[14]

He suggested a parochial committee be formed in each parish to assess the state of fever in the different streets and lanes, the condition of the poorer houses, and the nuisances such as dunghills and other filth. He further suggested that the parishioners should raise by voluntary assessment a sum that would pay the cost of whitewashing and cleansing the sewers and smaller lanes, removing pestiferous dunghills, washing bedclothes and purifying their narrow apartments, and so avert a further increase in fever. The Mayor, from personal experience, could confirm the filthy and unhealthy state of many of the houses in St. Mary's Parish. In some of the dwellings of the poor, the dunghills actually existed close to the beds of the inmates. The public were asked to help by procuring straw beds for the poor, ill with fever, 'the want of that most necessary article is in some degree a principal cause of producing contagion. One pound would provide straw for 20 families'. William Frazer of St. John's undertook to distribute the straw to the needy.[15]

The Sick Poor Fund was maintaining 844 people per week. The object of the charity was to relieve convalescent patients discharged from the fever hospital. In a report of the Sick Poor fund on 18th October Dr. William Geary said that no matter how big and well funded, a hospital is a temporary relief to its suffering inmates, and 'our Fever Hospital at this moment, presents very distressing features'. During convalescence, immediately following their discharge 'nature is denied suitable support'; as ex-patients were unable to procure the cheapest clothing, food, fuel or bedding. With the approach of winter he forecast that disease would increase.

Drought affected the crops in spring, which became scarce and proportionately dear during the summer and harvest. Oats in particular yielded a small quantity of straw which was the principal bedding of the poor. The small supply of potatoes, the main support of the peasantry and working classes, sold at sixpence per stone. He was surprised that:

> the poor, worn out by fatigue and hunger - exposed to every inclemency which the seasons offer, collecting themselves together at night in narrow rooms poorly supported with fuel - with scanty pittance - of deteriorated straw and in most instances no other clothing than the tattered shreds that served to cover them by day are not more frequently the victims of disease.[16]

The registered number of admissions into the Hospital for September was almost three times that of April. Dr. Geary believed that there would have been more relapse cases but for the existence of the "Sick Poor Fund", and the great advantages resulting from the distribution of wholesome provisions, oatmeal and new milk, to the convalescent fever patients. The Fund also held out a strong inducement to those with fever, to seek relief from the Hospital 'to which many hitherto offered insurmountable objections'. From 22 September to 5 November 1826, 2,768 individuals had been relieved, the daily average 62 people at a cost of three-half-pence each. In addition, they received large amounts of straw. The existence of the "Poor Fund" was very uncertain and totally dependent on the benevolent. Dr. William Geary, its treasurer, wanted to place the charity on a permanent footing, as the situation of those relieved was deplorable. He urged the compassionate to seriously consider the vast benefits they conferred through it and how deserving it was of their support. Advice to the public on how to prevent fever was recommended by Dr. Kingsley (Valley-House, Roscrea), to be posted up in every house and cabin, for constant reference in cases of necessity. Employment was to be given only to those who adhered strictly to the rules, as only by rigorous enforcement could the sole cause of infectious fever be removed. 'Comfortable clothing, wholesome food, and good lodgings, must eradicate every other cause, those however, can only be procured thro' the medium of constant employment given to the poorer classes of society.'[17] In November Dr. Geary reported a rapid increase of disease throughout the city since his nomination to the dispensary and he believed there were 'at least 150 now lying ill of fever in the Parishes of St. John and St. Michael, who cannot find admission to the Fever Hospital.'[18]

The crisis of 1826, while it was essentially agricultural, was exacerbated by a new factor. Economic union had recently followed on the political union of 1800 and the excess production of English textiles (mass produced) were dumped on the Irish market; to the detriment of the Irish textiles industry. The people of West Cork were in great distress and misery in April 1826. Young men in Bandon enlisted in the army or emigrated to America. In Roscarbery and Clonakilty many weavers were close to starvation as 'there was no demand for the produce of their looms, except at a price absolutely ruinous to themselves and their families'. Fever and dysentery followed.[19] The situation was similar in the Dublin liberties but was relieved somewhat in Drogheda, by the subscription of £200 from the King.[20] In the neighbourhood of Wexford town fever made frightful ravages among the poorer classes and Longford had fever of a most malignant kind. There were 918 people in the House of Industry in Cork and the Fever Hospital was crowded to excess. The funds of both were exhausted.[21] In the North, the demand for cotton ceased and about 10,000 Belfast weavers were out of work. In England mechanization caused problems for weavers also. There were riots in Bradford and weavers in Manchester accepted reduced wages to keep their jobs.[22]

In Limerick the potato crop was harvested in the greater part of the county in November and 'a finer produce has seldom been recollected'. Despite a temporary rise in admissions to St. John's Fever hospital early the following year (1827) the crisis had passed, for now.

Between 1821 and 1826 the amount of time a patient spent in hospital varied. In general, venereal patients stayed longer than fever patients. It was not unusual for venereally diseased patients to remain in hospital for several months and two women were inmates for 134 days and 162 days respectively. The routine may have been boring for these patients or some mental disorder may have been caused by their disease, to judge from the fact that eighteen venereally diseased patients, including a mendicant from the House of Industry were discharged for misconduct, (they soiled the walls), and another was discharged for 'irregularity'. All had been in hospital for between 2 to 6 weeks. The misconduct of another five discharged patients was not specified; one was a venereal patient, a groom from Roches Street, and another a 14 year old labourer's son with dysentery. Other patients were discharged because they did not have the disease they were thought to have when admitted. Twenty-six patients 'not having dysentery' - some were sent home the same day and others after several weeks. In one case the observation was more explicit "passing no blood and her case not being dysentery". Nineteen did not have fever (one of those had whooping cough), and sixteen had no venereal disease. Two inmates were discharged for not taking their medicine, and thereby exposing other patients to infection. Cross-infection was a real danger.

For one fever patient, 29 year old, Mary Buckley, an inmate for 86 days, it was a long wait for death. Patients who were dying when admitted were not always treated by the doctor in attendance so it was not so unusual that a 30 year old woman, died of dysentery after 3 days. What is unusual is the death of a 23 year old labourer's son who died of fever but was not seen by the doctor 'his case not being fever'.

Though generally well cared for in hospital, it must have been a cause of great hardship to a family when a parent was admitted, and frequently patients would not remain. A mason from Palmerstown who was found on admission to have dysentery, not fever, went home. Sixty-eight other patients, regardless of their disease, were discharged at their own request and sometimes that of their family and friends. A cured venereal patient went over the hospital wall at night, and another left by the door having been treated for dysentery for 91 days. Others required more comfort or privacy for example Mr. Loughlin, a 45 year old pensioner from Creagh Lane, admitted with fever, would not remain in the house because it was crowded, and a 46 year old labourer's wife from the Irishtown, would not remain because she could not have a room of her own! The hospital did not provide sanctuary and a 20-year old fever patient was taken prisoner by the police for attacking a counsellor.

Given that Limerick was a garrison town with a poor population, prostitution was inevitable, and the streets of Limerick in 1825 were crowded every night with prostitutes. The Magdalen Asylum was founded to protect female penitents 'seeking to return from the ways of vice'. It opened in March 1820 to every religious persuasion and had 34 inmates.[23] Patients came from the Magdalen Asylum and the House of Industry, and from other institutions to St. Johns. Venereal disease is an occupational hazard of prostitutes and many had venereal disease, especially mendicants, but most had fever. Not all admissions from these institutions were prostitutes. One patient who would not allow Dr. Vereker to examiner her, was discharged designated "a lunatic". Aged 15 - 30 years, they were labourer's wives, daughters, and a school- master's daughter who remained in hospital with fever for 119 days. Among those discharged to the House of Industry were, after only two days, a 40 year old woman who was admitted from the lying-in hospital with fever; another, aged 30, cured of venereal disease after 292 days; and an eighteen year old labourer cured of fever after 73 days. Two fever patients, one a mason, were discharged to the lunatic asylum.

Patients transferred from the lying-in-hospital, and the Alms House, and from the County Hospital, (a general medical and surgical hospital), to have their fevers attended to. Most were cured but some, like Mary Flannery, a twenty-seven year old labourer's wife, died of fever after 6 days. Three patients transferred from, St. John's to the County hospital; one with a gangrenous leg; a 14 year old orphan with fever, who got bed sores, having a been a patient in St. John's for 109 days; and a boy with pneumonia, having been treated for fever for 43 days. Two patients transferred to the lying-in hospital.

In 1826, nine 'poor scholars', all fever patients, stayed in St. John's hospital for periods of from 4 to 31 days. They ranged in age from 13 - 19 years. Five had no fixed abode and four gave County Limerick townlands as their address. In that same period there were 31 sailors and a sailor's wife, inmates of the hospital. Ten had addresses in Limerick. About two-thirds of sailors presented with fever, and the other third with venereal disease. The latter, a disproportionately high figure in terms of admissions, spent at least three weeks in hospital. Fever patients might stay as little as two days, or as much as eight or nine weeks. Ship-board fever was one of the most deadly and concentrated forms of typhus and the hospital provided an invaluable service in preventing its spread. In one relapse case, a castaway sailor spent 107 days in hospital. He recovered, but a thirty year old 'out of place' sailor, died of fever after 6 days, a relapse case. Joshua Brooks, a twenty-seven year old sailor, on the ship "Exchange", out of Baltimore, in America, was an inmate for 89 days before he died of venereal disease. Castaway sailors were not uncommon and while most patients were Irish, there were sailors from Wales, England, Scotland and America. Most sailors contributed financially towards the cost of their stay in hospital unless they were 'out of employ'. They usually paid £1 and the record would state whether it was British or Irish, but it could vary from eleven shillings and four pence halfpenny to £1.1.8 for no apparent reason. Payment was made on admission to the hospital.

Some other patients, (usually the venereal diseased), also contributed towards the cost of their stay and treatment in hospital. Servants and labourers usually paid ten shillings each, though they sometimes paid one pound. A small number of fever patients made a donation.

The staff of the hospital, particularly the nurses, suffered from, and in some cases died of fever. Those who survived the frequent epidemics increased their immunity but Mary Donohoe, aged 24, must have been susceptible. She had been ill with fever for 31 days in May 1822, and for 47 days in May 1823. She died of fever after 76 days in January 1825. Mary Leary, also a nurse, aged 42, died of fever after 16 days, in October 1826. It is striking how many were cured, even nurses who had repeated fevers didn't necessarily die of fever. Jane Brooks was infected six times with fever between 1822 - 1826. In 1821 three nurses are listed as being cured of fever, one suffering a further infection of fever in 1822, and Peggy Danaher aged 50 had dysentery for fifteen days. These were extraordinary women doing very difficult and dangerous work, and yet only two appear to have quit the job in the six year period under review. In all, fifteen nurses were ill with fever during this period. Not only were they in danger but their daughters were also victims of fever.

Notes

[1] St. John's Hospital Archive.
[2] Ó Gráda Ireland A New Economic History P.12.
[3] Geary, A Historical and Medical Report p 55.
[4] L.A. Clarkson and E.M Crawford, Life after Death: Widows in Carrick-on-Suir, 1799. In Margaret MacCurtain and Mary O'Dowd, (eds.). Women in Early Modern Ireland (Edinburgh 1991), p 241
[5] Griffin, An Inquiry into the Mortality p 308.
[6] Griffin, An Inquiry into the Mortality, p 318. The highest incidence of fever occurred in the ten-to-thirty age groups among patients admitted to Dublin hospitals during the period 1813 to 1818, p 126 'Typhus in Nineteenth-Century Ireland' E. M. Crawford. In Greta Jones and Elizabeth Malcolm, (eds.) Medicine, Disease and the State in Ireland, 1650-1940, (Cork 1999).
[7] C. E. Rosenberg, Explaining Epidemics and Other Studies in the History of Medicine; (Cambridge 1992), pp 10, 11, 14, 21, 25-26, 45.
[8] Quoted by Ó Gráda in Ireland A New Economic History P. 93.
[9] Ó Gráda Ireland A New Economic History Pp.85-86. Pp.90-94.
[10] Wilde, Report upon the Tables of Deaths, p xxiii.
[11] St. John's Hospital Archive.
[12] The Limerick Chronicle 4 March 1826
[13] The Limerick Chronicle 6 September 1826
[14] The Limerick Chronicle 9 September 1826
[15] Ibid.
[16] The Limerick Chronicle October 18, 1826.
[17] The Limerick Chronicle October 21, 1826.
[18] The Limerick Chronicle November 11, 1826.
[19] The Limerick Chronicle 12 April 1826.
[20] The Limerick Chronicle April 29 and May 13
[21] The Limerick Chronicle December 2, 1826.
[22] The Limerick Chronicle May 13 1826.
[23] The Limerick Chronicle 2 February 1825.

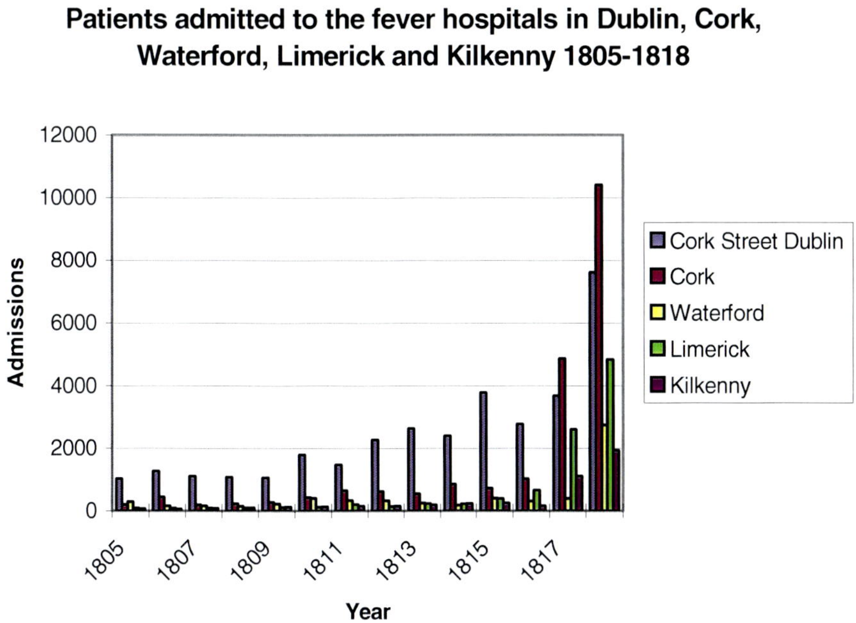

Fig. 3 Admissions to St. John's hospital were so great that to relieve the pressure a temporary hospital was set up nearby in The square on January 11th 1818. This hospital admitted 1,697 patients – 1,295 patients were admitted in 355 days. It closed on April 20th 1819.

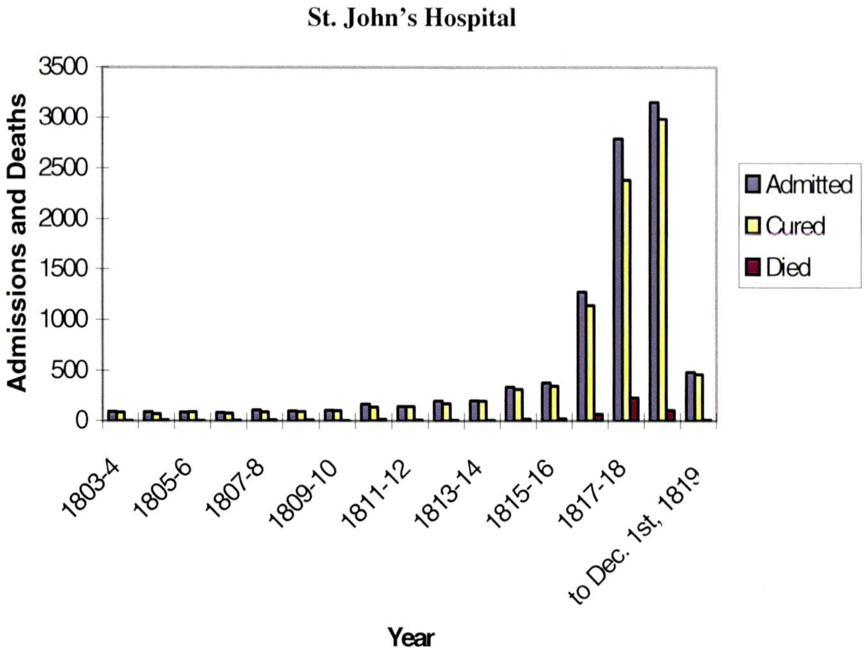
St. John's Hospital
Admissions and Deaths
3500
3000
2500
2000
1500
1000
500
0
Admitted
Cured
Died
1803-4
1805-6
1807-8
1809-10
1811-12
1813-14
1815-16
1817-18
to Dec. 1st, 1819
Year

Fig. 5.

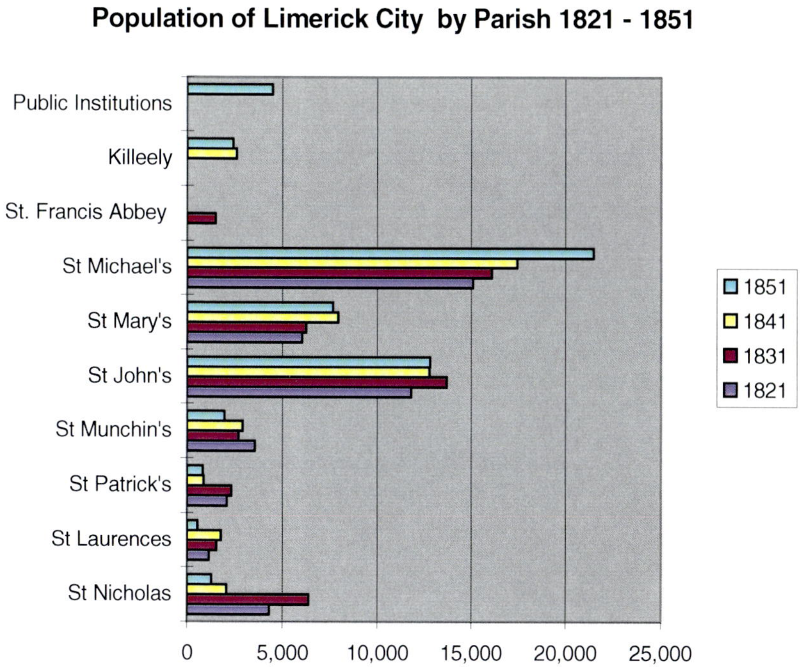
Population of Limerick City by Parish 1821 - 1851
Public Institutions
Killeely
St. Francis Abbey
St Michael's
St Mary's
St John's
St Munchin's
St Patrick's
St Laurences
St Nicholas
0
5,000
10,000
15,000
20,000
25,000
1851
1841
1831
1821

Fig. 6.

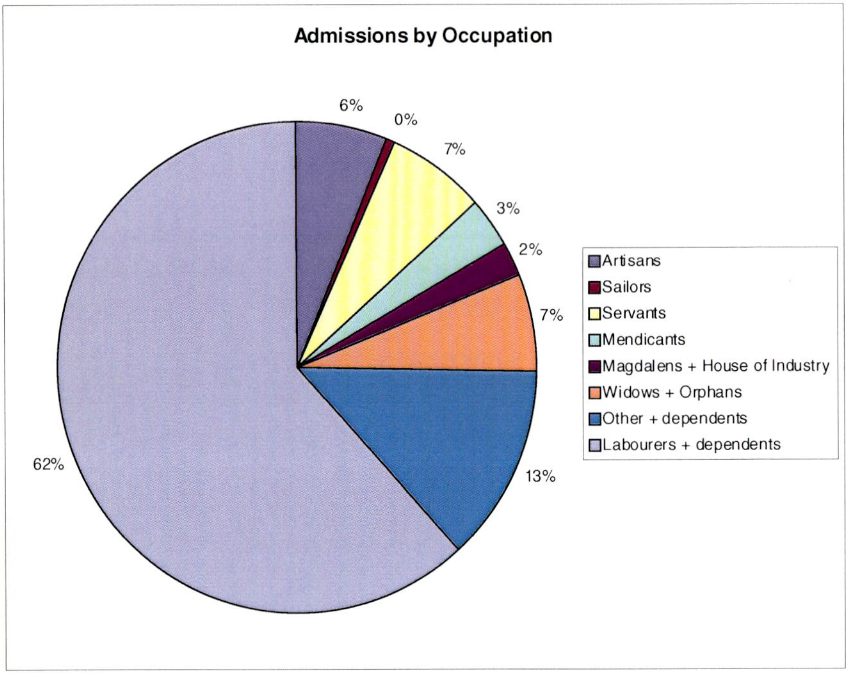

Fig. 7 St. John's Hospital Archive.

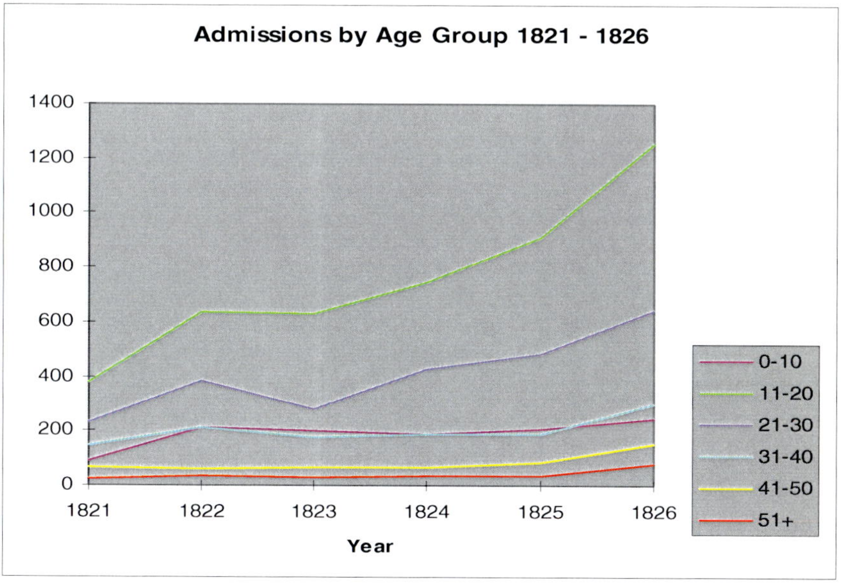

Fig. 8 St. John's Hospital Archive.

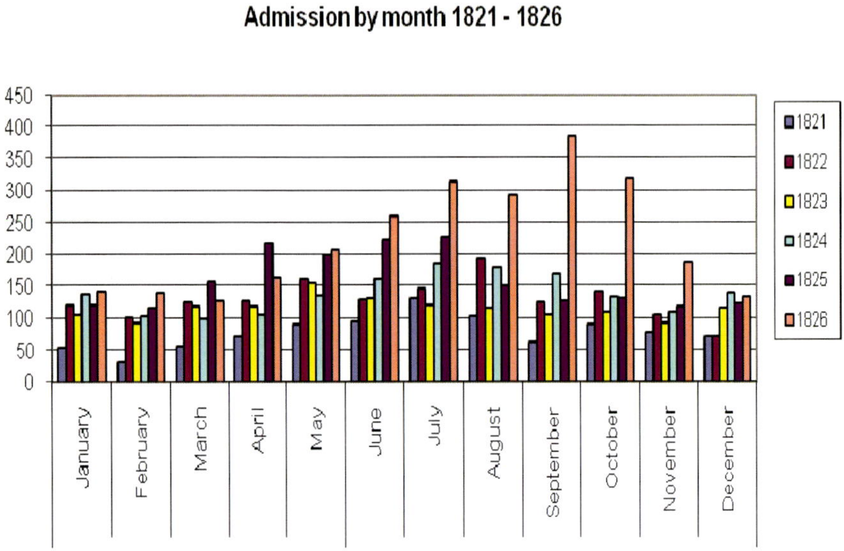

Fig. 9 St. John's Hospital Archive.

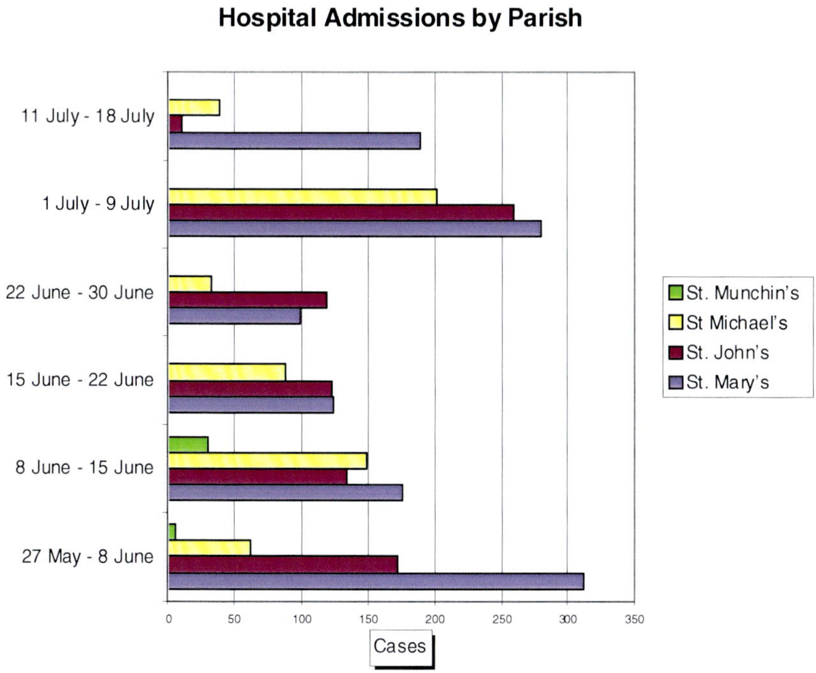

Fig. 10 Historical Records of the Existence and Progress of Cholera in the City of Limerick.

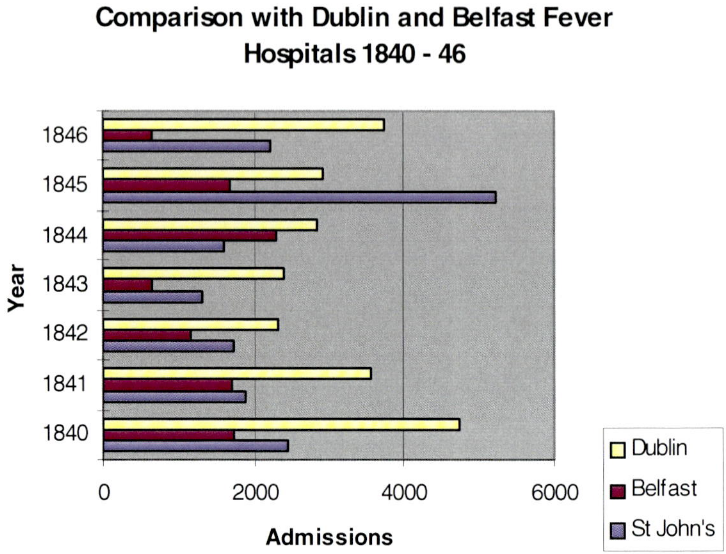

Fig. 11 St. John's Hospital Archives

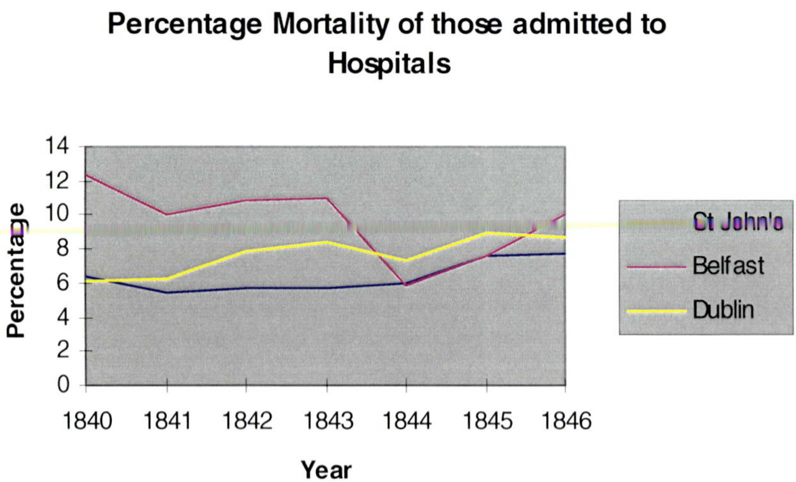

Fig. 12 St. John's Hospital Archives.

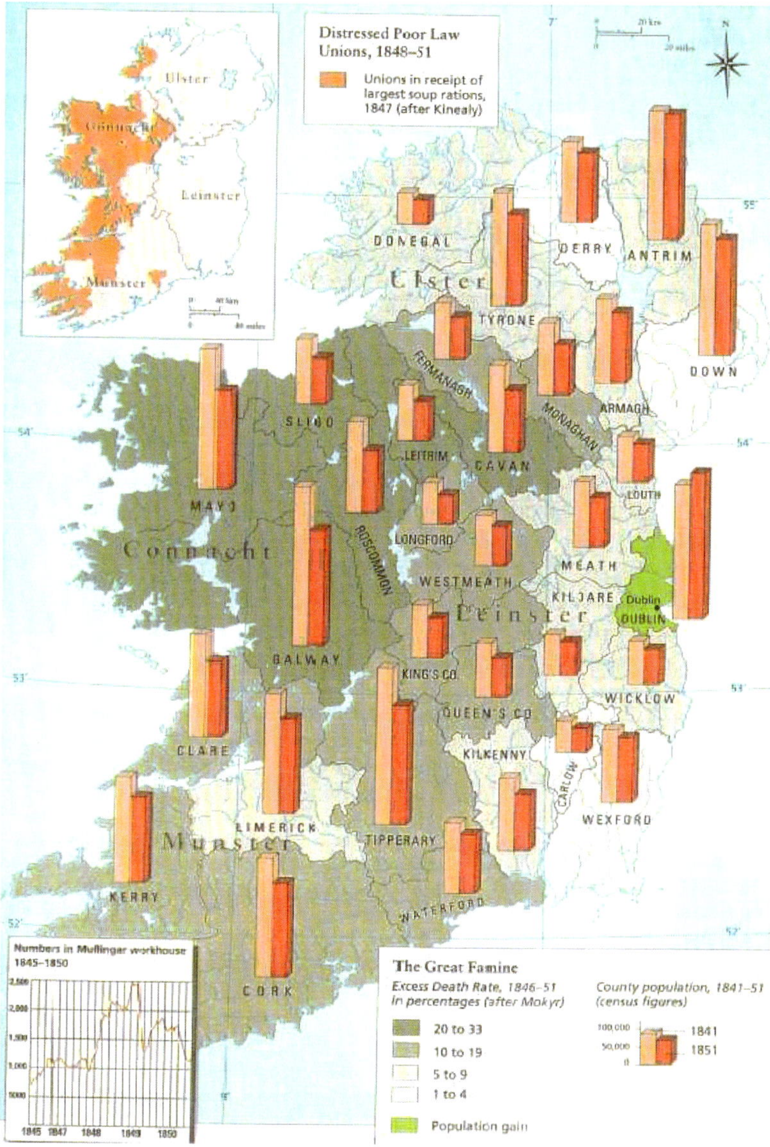

Fig. 13. It is clear from the above map that Limerick city was adjacent to some of the worst affected poor law unions.

CHAPTER FOUR

CHOLERA 1832

Cholera is a bacterial disease that affects the intestinal tract. Six worldwide outbreaks were documented between 1817 and 1911 that resulted in hundreds of thousands of deaths. Cholera was known for centuries in India and with the opening up of world trade routes in the nineteenth century, and the increase in Muslim and Hindu pilgrimages, it spread throughout the world. The second pandemic of cholera swept across Europe from Asia in 1824, reaching England in 1831. The germ is passed in the stools and is spread by eating or drinking food or water contaminated by fecal waste of an infected person. This occurs where adequate water supplies and proper sewage disposal are lacking. The symptoms include copious, painless, watery diarrhea, vomiting and rapid dehydration. Fever is usually absent.[1] Limerick city was aware of the existence of cholera in Europe, from the newspaper reports, but nothing was done until alarming accounts were received from Sunderland. The disease reached Ireland in April, 1832 making its first appearance in Cork and Dublin, with many fatalities.[2] So many poor and destitute people as well as whole families were swept away, during the epidemic of 1832 and 1833, and the disease caused such panic, that records of deaths from cholera are defective. With this caveat, Wilde, gives the number of deaths in Ireland from this disease as 25,378, and Limerick city as 1,105.[3] The higher incidence of cholera deaths in Ireland relative to Britain was a reflection of Irish poverty, according to Ó Gráda.[4]

On 25th April 1832 a meeting to discuss the situation was attended by the most influential inhabitants of the city, "and though met for benevolent purposes, was conducted in that spirit of acrimony and bad taste, which was quite at variance with the business of the day" [5]. However, The Central Board of Health was formed, and they in turn appointed Officers of Health in the parishes to establish a fund to meet the expenses of whitewashing the homes of the poor; sprinkling lime in the lanes and alleys, and to remove filth and nuisances from dwelling houses.[6] St. John's hospital was fitted out in the belief that it would accommodate any number of cholera cases that might arise.[7] The Liberties were called on, by the Mayor, to appoint Officers of Health in their parishes. The Board immediately applied to the Government for a loan of £500. The Lord Lieutenant urged caution in applying for funds as they would be ultimately borne by the County, and advised:

> It will be necessary to accompany the application for public aid by written documents, minutely detailing the number of persons suffering from Fever, and conveying the fullest information, with respect to the measures intended to be pursued, and the probable expenditure which they will occasion. ….vouchers must be kept of every item of expenditure, ….certified by five at least of the Members of the Board of Health.[8]

The Board received just £300, and with the Liberties free of taxation, there was not enough money to supply the poor with straw beds, fuel, food, or clothes or to open hospitals in each parish.[9]

On Tuesday, 8th May, 1832 the first case, that of a young man in St. Mary's parish, was diagnosed. This caused such alarm that within a short time the news spread throughout the City. The man was removed to St. John's hospital, where every antidote was administered, and he was soon restored to a state of comparative convalescence. There was much discussion among the physicians as to the nature of the man's illness but Dr. John Geary, gave his opinion that it was cholera in its milder form. The patient recovered but the case caused disquiet among the public, who doubted the honesty of the physicians and their knowledge of the disease, suggesting that this was an attempt to frighten people into getting cholera in order that the physicians would have something to do![10] The doctors themselves engaged in a public debate through the newspapers on the nature of the disease.[11] A meeting of invited physicians, chaired by Dr. Harding, was held at his house in Glentworth Street on May 12th, to consider the best arrangement for admitting and treating Spasmodic Cholera patients in the city hospitals. They decided to form a permanent Medical Board; that St. John's hospital with two physicians, should appoint Dr. William Geary as its Inspector; and that one senior physician, one inspector, and two junior physicians, would be sufficient to appoint to each of the other hospitals including the County hospital in the Island. The following evening, junior doctors held a meeting. They expressed themselves equally interested in the welfare of the sick poor, and complained of the private meeting that chose a Medical Board of Health when such a selection should have been made by the profession at large. They concluded:

> because the present self-constituted Medical Board can never prove an efficient assistant to the Board of Health, as we are justly resolved to accept no situation on their recommendation to report no cases through them, to hold no concert with them as a Board of Health, with respect to any measures necessary for the preservation of this City, but we will discharge the duties of humanity to every class of our fellow-Citizens, without reference to the existence of any such self-elected Body.[12]

On the 14th May, Denis Mullane, a corn-broker, in Boherbuoy, a less prosperous part of St. Michael's parish separated from Perry Square only by some waste ground, had been working in his garden all day. He was seized with severe spasms and stomach cramps. After lingering in the most agonizing pain for seven hours, he died at five o'clock next morning. Surgeon Barry was sent for and he called in Dr. John Geary, who concurred in his diagnosis of cholera. Several other physicians were called. The people of Boherbuoy were violently opposed to the visits of the physicians, but were calmed by the clergy, and the constant visits of the police. Immediately after the death of Mullane, the Officers of Health brought a coffin and hearse in order to have the remains removed to the churchyard, but friends, relations and neighbours of the deceased insisted on taking the body to Newcastle West. The rest of the family was removed. The house was fumigated and locked up, in an effort to contain the disease. But on the following day the sister-in-law of Mullane, was taken ill. The mob, frightened by the appearance of the 'Cholera Cot' attempted to break it, and beat the men who carried it. The 'Cholera Cot', which was used to transport the sick to hospital, consisted of a seven feet long wooden box, on four legs with two long poles for carrying. It contained a pallet to lie on, and a pair of blankets to cover the patient.[13]

The distrust of the Board of Health by the people was due to their reluctance to spend money, especially in St. Mary's parish, and the belief that the Board's real concern was to ward off the contagion from the "rich ones" of St. Michael's parish, (exempt from taxation by Act of Parliament, so they could not be called on to repay any portion of the £300 loan) and protecting the Liberties from taxation.[14] "Many of their discussions were marked by that local political bias, and those strong and party electioneering feelings which have proved the bane of this City for the last twenty years."[15] The Board was forced to act following the alarming outbreak of cholera in St. Mary's parish. Most of the population were paupers. No hospital had been fitted up, nor streets cleansed, nor houses whitened, except what had been done by the Local Officers. A handbill posted up by one of the assistant Officers of Health in that parish read

".....that the bodies of our abandoned poor must smoulder in destructive putrefaction, forsooth, because they died in some instances outside the Hospitals. Oh! shame on such degrading parsimony .....R.K.O'B."[16] On 15th May the Limerick Chronicle carried a request from the Board of Health for Medical practitioners disposed to offer their services at the several hospitals about to be established.[17] On May 26th, eleven people died of cholera, and terror and dismay spread through the city. Streets became deserted, as most shops and some commercial establishments closed, and business, both civil and military, was almost suspended. Workers were discharged, thereby adding to the poverty of the people. The courts and the Exchange remained closed for several days. No guard was mounted nor were the red-coats to be seen parading the streets, - not even a bugle was heard at noon, or tattoo at evening. Only the poor and needy, the benevolent and humane, and those who had to act officially towards the sick to create funds for the poor and the destitute, ventured out. Physicians advised people not to use fish of any sort, vegetables, spirituous or malt liquors, except brandy, and wine.[18]

The Mayor called a public meeting in June, for the purpose of creating, by voluntary subscription, a fund to open soup-kitchens, and supply bedding and clothes, to the destitute. A number of gentlemen afraid of catching the disease, sent their apologies, and said they would "do the same as their neighbours". The Mayor and several of those present spoke in favour of the motion. Mr. John Boyle, proprietor of the Cork Freeholder, denounced the course the Chairman and many of the preceding speakers were pursuing as irrelevant, since they would not agree to taxing the Liberties. Mr. James Morgan addressed the meeting and referred to the state of the Subscription List, "and dwelt, in no very measured but respectful terms, on the parsimony of Mr. Spring Rice, the Earl of Limerick, the Marquis of Lansdowne, the Lord Bishop of Limerick, and many others." The meeting, though poorly attended, raised over £300.[19]

On 4th June the streets of the different parishes were strewn with lime to purify the air and sewers. Four days later the Central Board appointed grave diggers for the different churchyards in the city and Liberties. Some men were in such dread of the disease, that in many instances women were compelled to take part in carrying coffins to the grave. On one occasion a young girl was seen moving towards the churchyard holding a coffin on her head containing the remains of her little brother, with no one to help her. Notices were posted up throughout the city advising the public not to attend funerals, or wakes of patients who had died of cholera.[20]

St. John's was the first hospital in Limerick fitted up for cholera patients. The beds were arranged in three rows along the walls. When it first opened, each of the patients had a nursetender to wait on them, and they were attended by the physicians, clergymen, the officers of health and the apothecaries, in a hospital run with order and precision. The hospital was well supplied with "good prime beef, bread, tea, milk, whey, wine and brandy which was dealt out to the sick with unsparing hand, as far as was consistent with their situation." Friends of cholera victims were invited to visit the sick, and brought favourable reports back to neighbours, so that new cases went at once to St. John's hospital.[21]

Bishop Ryan would not allow the College in Park, a townland within the municipal boundary, where the Bishop resided, to be used as a temporary hospital for St. Mary's parish, so the Ladies of St. Clare's Convent and Father Enraght provided the school-house. The nunnery hospital, as it was known, opened on the 30th May. Benefactors supplied old bedsteads, bedding, bathing-pans, and other necessities of a temporary hospital. Male and female patients shared the same ward.[22] One Surgeon Peppard was appointed inspector of the nunnery hospital. His interference in the treatment of the patients was resented by the attending physicians, the officers of health, the nursetenders and the frightened patients. Two died as a result – one he bled too much and the other he overdosed with medicine. Father Enraght on behalf of the others rebuked the surgeon who became outraged. When he calmed down Peppard said he would resign, but instead complained to the Board about Enraght. He got no support from the Bishop or the other doctors, but "Enraght was right and the people knew it and would stand by him."[23] Peppard was next appointed, through the influence of one Dickson, a relative on the management board, to St. John's hospital, where he was as obnoxious as he had been at the nunnery. Dickson too was a difficult character; having drink taken, he called unexpectedly to the nunnery hospital and ordered some of the bedsteads to be taken to the convalescent hospital in Clare Street. In strong language he was ordered to leave the house by the local officers.[24]

The hired nursetenders in the nunnery, owing to inebriety, were dismissed and were replaced by the Magdalens. "These humane creatures did their duty very becomingly and tenderly, which could not be otherwise while under the superintendence of Miss Reddan and Miss Bridgeman, the conducting matrons." Hospital visitors sometimes remained up all night offering relief and consolation.[25] Contempt was all one unnamed visitor to the hospital had for the Central Board of Health;

> they are indebted for nothing that could give them assistance, but what they considered their right, and whatever they could force. They cannot discover why their claims on the Board of Health were refused for coffins, and other means of interment for persons who died outside the walls of the hospital - persons who had received every assistance in their power, the hospital at the time being literally crowded.[26]

On the 6th June - twenty-six people died within the previous twenty-four hours, due to insufficient liquid, allegedly as a result of the parsimony, of the Central Board, in refusing funds to the Local Officers. Many of the cholera victims were interred in the nunnery burial ground, there being no friend or relative to claim them. The disease became virulent from May 26, when several cases in the parishes of St. Mary and St. John, proved fatal. The average number of deaths per day was 16, and most of those took place in the nunnery hospital. The disease having greatly increased, especially, in St. Mary's parish, Barrington's hospital opened on 12 June, to accommodate them. The following day it became very fatal in the parish of St. Michael, especially in Little Anne Street and Market Alley, and both rich and poor died. At this period private deaths averaged one to four of the hospital reports. By the end of June deaths were averaging 154 each week. After raging for just over a month cholera abated in the parishes of St. Mary and St. Munchin, and on June 20, the nunnery hospital closed; subsequent cases were sent to Barrington's hospital. The beds were removed to the Lancastrian School-house in Clare Street, which was converted into a convalescent hospital.[27]

Barrington's hospital, in St. Mary's parish, was built and endowed by the Barrington family as a general hospital for the poor of Limerick City in 1829. On average it dressed 10,950 minor accidents annually and prescribed for 20,000 sick poor, and could accommodate 100 patients.[28] When the influx to the nunnery hospital became greater than they could deal with, the Board of Health applied for the use of Barrington's Hospital, which was readily granted by the Governors and Proprietors. The patients then in Barrington's were transferred to the County Infirmary, and the wards were immediately fitted up and opened for cholera patients, on the 5th June. It was full in a very short time. The internal arrangements of this hospital far excelled those of St. John's, owing to the rules of the house devised by the committee, and required only an increase of physicians, apothecaries, and nursetenders. The patients were well cared for but admittance through the front entrance on George's Quay was deemed likely to give offence to the gentry on Charlotte's Quay, and those adjacent to the hospital. The Board of Health ordered that the Cholera Cot should be admitted through the back gate in Mary Street and that the dead should be taken out by the same passage. This created fear and resentment against the doctors and the General Board, but the people of Mary Street became reconciled to the arrangement rather than disturb the peace of the dying.[29]

In St. Michael's parish the Christian Brothers gave the use of their school-house at Upper William Street, for conversion into a cholera hospital on 2nd May. The attendants were not as active as they should have been, and a few of the Magdalens were brought from the nunnery hospital.[30]

The Officers of Health for St. Munchin's Parish, had an old house on the North Strand, commonly known as the "Rose Tavern", converted into a temporary hospital, which operated from the 5th to the 22nd June. Here too the nursetenders were a problem. However, it was closed by order of the Board, against the will of the entire population of the two Parishes.[31] The people of St. Mary's complained that the appearance of the Cholera cot created much fear; it was unreasonable to drag patients from Thomondgate, a distance of one mile through Mary Street when there was a hospital already fitted up in that parish. The Board refused to reopen it. The Mayor, the Hon. J.P. Vereker, delivered the answer at a meeting between Board and people. A placard was posted up through the Parish of St. Mary on the morning of the meeting, as follows:

> Caution! - Parishioners of St. Mary, - It pleased Providence that you should be sorely afflicted with this destructive malady that rages so furiously through our City. Many a widow and many an orphan left unsheltered and unprovided for. Is it not enough for you to bear your own sorrows and sufferings from this awful visitation of Divine Will, but must your hospital (in the centre of your families) be made a receptacle for the patients of every other infected parish, while they can be provided at home. No, neither does necessity, nor moral, nor religious obligations demand it, but forsooth to spare a paltry trifle - therefore RESIST IT quietly and peacefully resist it, for "SELF PRESERVATION IS THE FIRST PRINCIPLE OF NATURAL LAW". Allow no cases of CHOLERA from other Districts to be carted into your parish!!![32]

The Mayor told the people that the Board would not comply with their request, and that any resistance to the introduction of patients from Thomondgate would be met by force. He suggested, however, that they send their Officers of Health as a deputation to the Board, where he believed they would get a favourable hearing. The request to keep Thomondgate hospital open would have been granted but for the opposition of Bishop Ryan, who claimed that every other parish in the

Liberties would demand the same privilege, and there were neither funds nor physicians available. He refused his consent and insisted that the laws be enforced. Speaking on behalf of the people, the Rev. Mr. Enraght spoke for the application. The Bishop became angry, and assuming a more authoritative air challenged Mr. Enraght. The exchange that took place left the deputation and a number of Protestant gentlemen equally disgusted with the Bishop's conduct. The meeting would have broken up in disorder but the Mayor terminated the proceedings, by requesting the deputation to use their influence with the people, and point out to them the impossibility of keeping Thomondgate hospital open.[33]

In the garrison, out of 132 cases, since the 27th May, 12 men, 2 women, and one child were reported to have died of cholera. A portion of St. Munchin's church-yard was allotted for the remains of the military that died in this garrison. The grave-digger acknowledged that he had interred nearly thirty people from the New Barracks within a six week period, but could not say whether all died of cholera. Since the survival rate was so much higher here, it was assumed that the mode of treatment adopted by Doctor O'Callaghan, the Medical Officer in charge of the Military hospital, differed essentially from that of the city hospitals. He complied with the urgent pleas of several Boards of Health for his mode of treatment, which became practice in local hospitals.[34]

The total number of hospital cases of cholera was 2,602 and hospital deaths numbered 953.[35] Though not contagious, it was believed, fear was a predisposing cause. Catholic priests seldom got cholera though they constantly visited the infected habitations of the poor and spent hours with them. A doctor and two apothecaries from the country died of cholera, but none of the city physicians succumbed to the disease.[36]

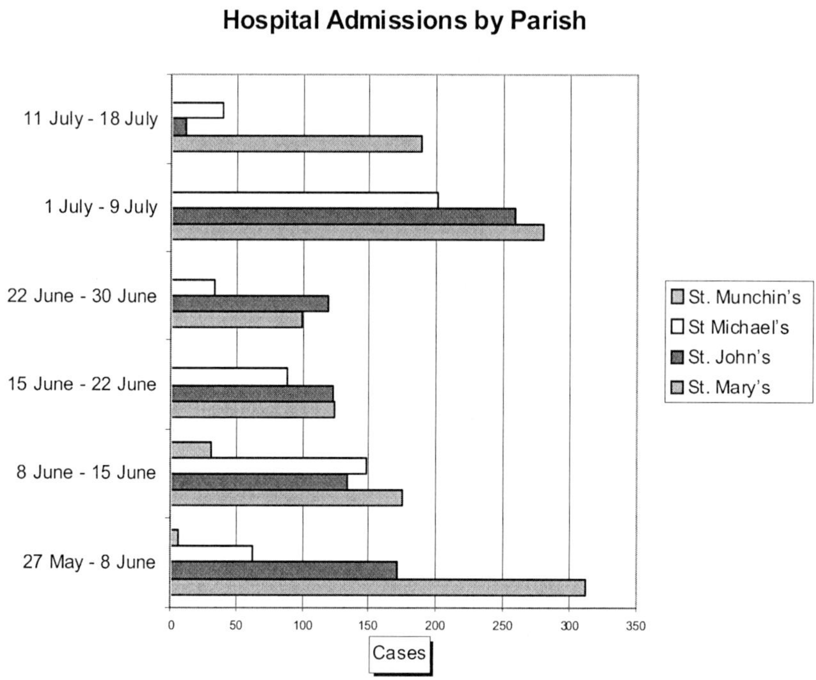

Fig. 10 Historical Records of the Existence and Progress of Cholera in the City of Limerick. See Centrefold for this image in colour.

From 1826 the citizens of Limerick paid between £4-5,000 per annum for an unfiltered water supply. Work to provide the city with clean water began in 1834. Two tanks were placed about a mile from the city, at Cromwell's Fort, near Gallow's Green. The water was raised 72 feet above the river by two 20 horse power steam-engines.[37] The need for an uninterrupted water supply was to extinguish fires[38] as the causes of cholera were unknown until 1880s.

Notes

[1] Porter, Cambridge Illustrated History of Medicine p.41. World Health Organisation factsheet.
[2] Historical Records of the Existence and Progress of Cholera in the City of Limerick, During the Months of May and June, 1832. Deane, Limerick 1832. Pp.7-11. (hereafter Historical Records of Cholera in the City of Limerick)
[3] Census of Ireland 1841. Report upon the Tables of Deaths by Wilde, Esq. Dublin Castle 1843.P.ii, Pp. xix-xx.
[4] Ó Gráda, Ireland A New Economic History p. 98
[5] Historical Records of Cholera in the City of Limerick, P.11
[6] Historical Records of Cholera in the City of Limerick. P.10.
[7] Historical Records of Cholera in the City of Limerick P.14
[8] Historical Records of Cholera in the City of Limerick. Pp.12-13. O'Brien, State Intervention and the Medical Relief p. 202 claims that grants were 'traded' for fully completed information returns during the epidemic.
[9] Historical Records of Cholera in the City of Limerick. P.25. O'Brien, State Intervention and the Medical Relief p. 202 – the cost of fighting the epidemic was spread over the county rather than 'fall upon single parishes'.
[10] Historical Records of Cholera in the City of Limerick. Pp.14-16.
[11] The Limerick Herald 10 May 1832, The Limerick Chronicle 12 May, 1832.
[12] Historical Records of Cholera in the City of Limerick, Pp.19-21.
[13] Historical Records of Cholera in the City of Limerick, Pp.21-24
[14] Historical Records of Cholera in the City of Limerick, P.26. O Gráda, Ireland A New Economic History p.98. When cholera struck in 1832, causing widespread panic, the better-off were told that their best safeguard was to help the poor.
[15] Historical Records of Cholera in the City of Limerick, P.27.
[16] Historical Records of Cholera in the City of Limerick, Pp.27-28.
[17] Historical Records of Cholera in the City of Limerick, P.28.
[18] Historical Records of Cholera in the City of Limerick, Pp.30-32.
[19] Historical Records of Cholera in the City of Limerick, Pp.33-38
[20] Historical Records of Cholera in the City of Limerick, Pp.68-69.
[21] Historical Records of Cholera in the City of Limerick, Pp.38-40.
[22] Historical Records of Cholera in the City of Limerick, Pp.40-41.
[23] Historical Records of Cholera in the City of Limerick, Pp.49-53.
[24] Historical Records of Cholera in the City of Limerick, Pp.53-55.
[25] Historical Records of Cholera in the City of Limerick, Pp.42-43.
[26] Historical Records of Cholera in the City of Limerick, Pp.42.
[27] Historical Records of Cholera in the City of Limerick, Pp.43-45.
[28] Minutes Barrington's Hospital 25 November 1846.
[29] Historical Records of Cholera in the City of Limerick, Pp.45-47.
[30] Historical Records of Cholera in the City of Limerick, Pp.47-48.
[31] Historical Records of Cholera in the City of Limerick, P.48
[32] Historical Records of Cholera in the City of Limerick, P.56.
[33] Historical Records of Cholera in the City of Limerick, Pp.55-59.

[34] Historical Records of Cholera in the City of Limerick, Pp.63-65.
[35] Historical Records of Cholera in the City of Limerick, Pp.70-71.
[36] Historical Records of Cholera in the City of Limerick, P.61.
[37] Lewis, History and Topography of Limerick p 123
[38] A Scheme for a Water Supply to the City of Limerick by M.A. Hennessy C.E. published by J.F. O'Gorman, Limerick 1879. P. 128 Ferrar, The History of Limerick p 128 Fire consumed more than 80 thatched houses in St. Francis's Abbey in 1755.

CHAPTER FIVE

THE FAMINE AND AFTER 1840 - 1890

Population increase was most rapid among the indigent classes and small tenant farmers, and in the poorer districts of Munster and Connacht. About two-thirds of a population of over 8 million in 1841 depended on the land for a living, and it could not bear the increasing pressure. Competition for land led to inflated rents and a rapid reduction in the rewards for labour. Absentee landlords, continuous sub-division of already small holdings, and post 1815, a steady trend from labour-intensive tillage to pastoral farming were major problems. Towns swarmed with beggars as no industries existed to absorb the increase in the population. Not only did Ireland (except for east Ulster)[1] fail to undergo an industrial revolution but it actually de-industrialized. The invention of the power-loom in 1785, and the development of steam power mechanized textile spinning, and by the 1820s – weaving. Ireland's resources of coal and iron, so necessary in the steam age, were limited, and importing them added to production costs. Tariffs which had protected Irish industry from English competition were abolished in 1824, increasing the distress and unemployment as cottage industries gave way to mass-produced imports. The home market could not compete with cheaper British imports, but the full effect would not be felt until the railways had formed a network throughout Ireland after the Famine.

A royal commission had recommended the construction of an elaborate network of railways in Ireland, but the Whig Government was unwilling to encroach in an area of free enterprise,[2] until the Famine crisis when the State invested £600,000 with railway companies after a Railway Act passed in 1847. Railways would have been vital in food distribution, helping to improve nutrition by delivering foods quickly and widely. In Ireland the standard of living declined appreciably in the 1820s and 1830s. The decay of manufacturing industry increased the burdens borne by the Irish taxpayer. There was a duty on Irish property owners to support Irish paupers, but it ignored the fact that many Irish estates were already too heavily encumbered with debt to honour this obligation.[3] The poor existed on the single staple food, the potato, - a standard of life at the hunger level. Only the potato could have met the needs of the expanding population; easy to grow and yielding a heavier food crop than any other in proportion to the area it occupied. Potatoes have a high calorific value per unit of land, which, in addition to filling stomachs, are an important source of vitamins (especially ascorbic acid) and minerals. Scurvy is a vitamin C deficiency which causes spongy, bleeding gums, old wounds open, and then death occurs. It added to the miseries of the Famine when the potato crop failed, because the grains sent to relieve the plight of the hungry did not contain this essential vitamin.[4] The potato crop could not be relied on, and the failures of 1817, and 1821 brought State grants in the form of public works schemes in an effort to relieve the misery. Bad harvests and high rents caused social tensions which could not always be contained and the government enforced the law of the land. The fall in grain prices made it difficult for farmers to pay their rent and evictions became more common in the 1820s and 1830s.[5] There was no safety margin and every bad harvest threatened a great part of the population with starvation, but it was disease rather than hunger that killed most people during the Famine.[6]

How well did St. John's rise to this challenge? In November 1845 the hospital committee noted with alarm the extent and continuing increase of fever in the district, especially since the potato crop was threatened by blight throughout the country. The potato crop was heavy in 1845 but only one-sixth was dug, in September and October, before the blight struck. The late crop, which is taken up in December and January, was diseased and, on opening the pits it was often found, that the potatoes had become a mass of rottenness.[7] A wet spring and humid summer brought total failure of the 1846 crop. Previous epidemics alerted the hospital management to the fact that fever increased as food became scarce. The Protestant Bishop of Limerick, writing to the Earl of Clare on 10 September 1850, claimed that "St. John's can challenge comparison with any similar institution in the kingdom." This would appear to be true from the Returns for 1840 - 46 which compares St. John's with Dublin's Cork Street and Belfast Fever Hospitals. In these years admission figures for Dublin, as the larger city, are higher, as one would expect, with the exception of 1845 when St. John's intake is almost double that of Dublin. What is more surprising is that the average rate of mortality was lowest in St. John's at 6.38 per cent, followed by Dublin at 7.66 per cent and Belfast at 9.67 per cent. Limerick was a city of great poverty while the Belfast district had nineteen factories spinning yarn by 1841, and would have had greater resources for caring for their sick.

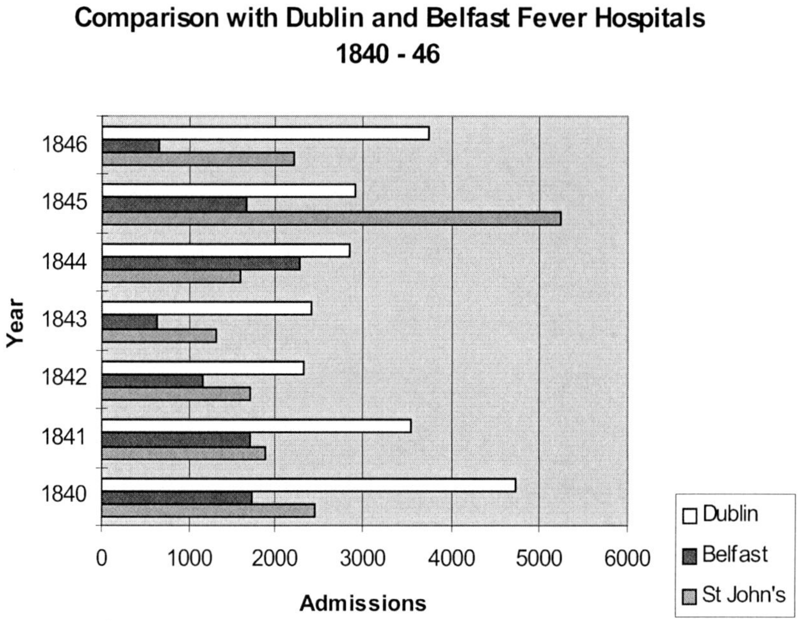

Fig. 11 St. John's Hospital Archives. See Centrefold for this image in colour.

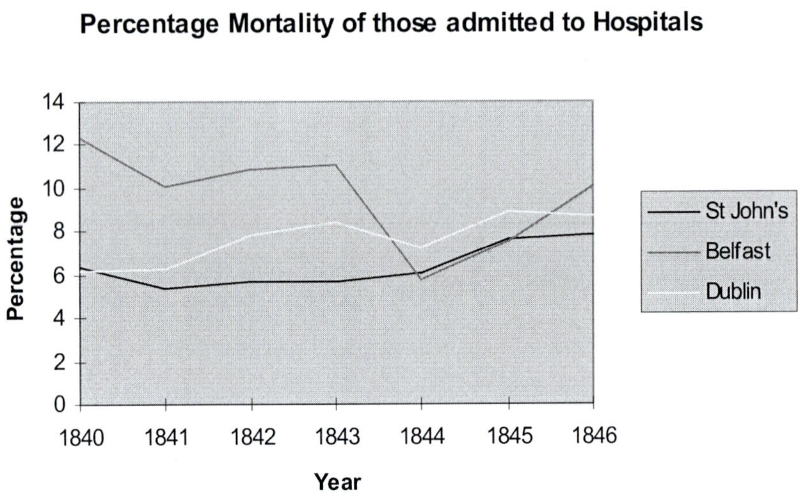

Fig. 12 St. John's Hospital Archives. See Centrefold for this image in colour.

Fever reached unprecedented heights with nearly 5,000 admissions and 344 deaths in eleven months, of 1845, and represented only half of the total number suffering from fever in the city. The previous highest figure for any year had been 3,499 admissions. Yet there were only 1,168 paupers in the Limerick workhouse which could accommodate 1,600, in November 1845. The funds of the fever hospital were nearly exhausted. An appeal was launched on the 19th November, for contributions to aid the sick and suffering poor. All classes were in danger of getting fever but particularly the parishes of the Old Town – St. John's, St. Mary's and St. Munchin's. A committee was set up which included the Mayor, and Protestant and Catholic clergymen to open a subscription list and consider what measures should be taken to prevent the spread of the disease. At a meeting of the Board of Barrington's hospital in December 1845, it was decided that the wards which had been used for the Mont de Piété, a charitable pawn office, 'be appropriated for the reception of convalescent patients discharged from the Fever Hospital', and Mr. Monsell be requested to confer with the Board of Guardians 'as to the desireableness of immediately purchasing such proportion of the bedding as may be ultimately required for the new hospital now in progress of erection at the work house'.[8] Admissions fell to 2,204 during 1846, the year that the Limerick Conference of the St. Vincent de Paul Society was established. The fall-off in admissions was due to a decrease in fever, which according to Dr. Gelston,[9] was a result of the change in the diet of the poor from the potato to imported grain (maize). When the watery potato was the only food of the poor, diseases of the digestive tract were most frequent and these were characterised by irritation of the mucous membrane of the alimentary canal, - 'one cause of the great fatality of typhus fever in this county'. The new Whig Government's response to the Famine was to introduce a number of Public works schemes to provide employment, so people could earn money and buy food. By January 1847, 31,506 people were employed daily on public works in the County and, 690 in the City of Limerick.[10] At the same time, "many of the poor people from the county were coming into the city. The streets literally swarm with country paupers".[11] Dr. Gelston adds 'in the entire of the past year, each month shows a gradual decrease in the number of applications for admission' [to the Fever hospital]. The fall-off in the number seeking medical relief was also observed in the City Dispensary, and in the hospitals attached to the county and city gaols.[12] Meat, milk and bread were the victuals of St. John's Hospital and not yellow meal. When funds were exhausted, relief work was phased out. The Society of Friends operated their soup kitchens from Barrington's Hospital, which was in a very embarrassed state financially and was compelled to request a small monthly rent. Another wing was used as a lying-in hospital and the ladies committee agreed to vacate the premises on repayment of £70 which they had laid out on the house.[13] Auxiliary workhouses opened in the summer of 1847 to take the excess from the main workhouse where mortality was very high; the majority of deaths took place immediately after admission. The Limerick Poor Law Guardians met on 20th September, 1847, and appointed a Committee, which sought the co-operation of Barrington's Hospital and St. John's Fever Hospital. The Governors were asked to assign the Hospitals to the Poor Law Guardians to serve as Union Hospitals for Poor Persons affected with fever or other contagious disease. The management of Barrington's agreed to hand over the Hospital on payment of £250 rent. The request was rejected by St. John's, as the management wished to continue to provide accommodation for poor persons not admissible to a Union Fever Hospital. They did however agree a rate per head per week for the maintenance of the lock cases in the workhouse.

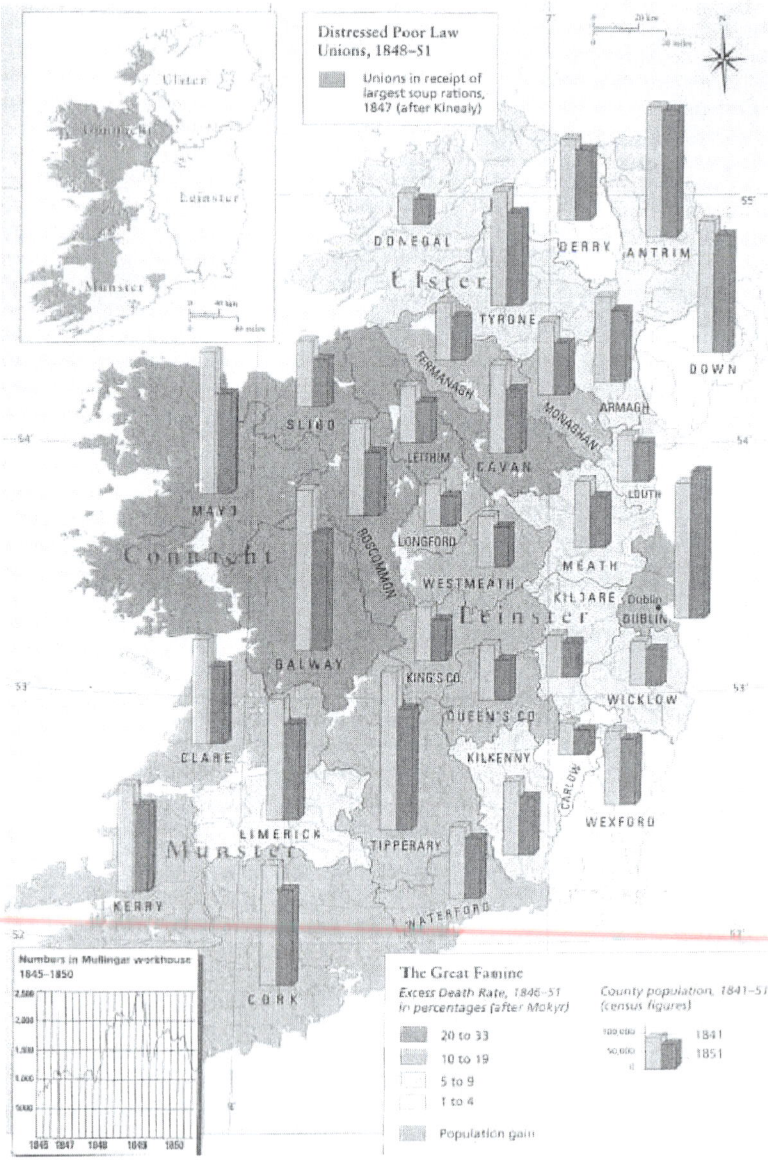

Fig. 13. It is clear from the above map that Limerick city was adjacent to some of the worst affected poor law unions. See Centrefold for this image in colour.

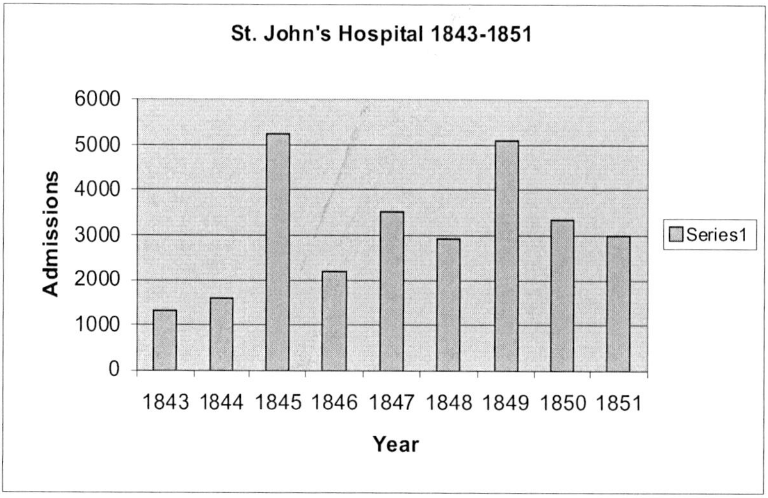

Fig.14 Limerick Its History and Antiquities.

The number of admissions increased in 1847 by more than a third to 3,525, though significantly less than the peak of 1845. Sixteen extra nurses were employed and the price of provisions was high due to the Famine. Expenditure in 1845 was extremely high but was matched by income with a small balance in hand at the end of the year.[14] While it was not unusual for St. John's to exceed its budget most years, income was down in 1847 and having paid the sum of £1,402 to creditors, £1,172 was still owing on 5th January 1848. This was excessive. The exhausted state of the funds forced the Committee to limit admissions to less than a quarter of its capacity. Unlike previous epidemics, the pattern of admissions to St. John's, therefore, bears no relation to the general incidence of fever. In May it was necessary to insert a notice in the Limerick Chronicle advising the public that admissions had been so great (601 in May), that they could not meet the demand for accommodation and in consequence admission would be limited to inhabitants of the city and county from this date. Only the increased contributions from the County and City Grand Juries made it possible to keep the hospital open for the reception of patients.

> This state of the funds, and consequent inability to afford the *accustomed unrestricted relief*, is a subject for grave consideration, when we reflect that the prospects of the Harvest are not such as to give a reasonable hope of any diminution of the Epidemic Fever which always exists in this

district, and which is ever aggravated by the distress and privation of the humbler classes.[15]

Dr. William Geary's political activism, as a member of the Young Irelanders, raised the ire of one cleric, the Administrator of St. John's [Cathedral], who in the letters column of The Limerick Reporter Newspaper of 1847 wrote 'not one voice was raised against the resolution withdrawing confidence from Dr. Geary[16] on political grounds'. However, a rebuttal in the form of a letter dated 14 October 1847 appeared in the same paper from the P.P. of St. Patrick's, showing that normal factionalism persisted even during the famine.

St. John's was constantly in financial difficulties. At a meeting on 22 August 1848 the committee decided that though the hospital was in a fitting condition to accommodate 200, no more than 31 cases would be treated in a day for the next 8 months, due to lack of funds. In an effort to secure funding, the committee asked the Board of Guardians, of the Limerick Union, to consider engaging 100 beds for fever cases only, on the understanding that the cost of the patients be in proportion to the weekly expenditure of the institution and no higher. This proposal was accepted, as fever had broken out and begun to spread in the workhouse to a serious extent, and all fever cases occurring in the workhouse from 31 August 1848 - 24 March 1849 were sent to St. John's Hospital. The Relieving Officer at the same time sent fever patients to St. John's but didn't feel it necessary to draw the Commissioner's attention to the permanent advantages derived from this arrangement. The ratio of deaths to admissions of the fever cases rose in this period to 1:16, and 1:49 of venereal cases. The Poor Law Commissioners in Dublin wrote on 3 August 1850 advising the Clerk of the Limerick Union that the Relieving officer's provisional power under section 7 of the Irish Poor Relief extension Act

> 'does not authorize him to send a person to the Saint John's Fever Hospital and that no person can be sent there except from the workhouse…..'

The Limerick Union comprised the City of Limerick, east county Limerick, and a large portion of south-east Clare, with a workhouse in Limerick city.[17] There were three workhouses in the county, namely Rathkeale, Kilmallock and Newcastle West.

Each district bore the cost of their own poor in the workhouse, and the Union at large paid the costs of poor people with no fixed abode. The city members of the Board of Guardians, attended meetings, which were held in the workhouse, more regularly than the rural members and had no difficulty in charging a high proportion of applicants for relief to the Union at large, much to the annoyance of the rural members. The City division contributed 46% of the inmates, with most of the city poor being migrants from the countryside.[18]

There were 1,136 inmates in the Limerick workhouse on 1st January 1845, rising to 1,290 by January 1846. By March the number was 2,512. Built originally to accommodate only 1,600, additions were made yearly, and by the end of the famine there were three separate buildings.[19]

When the head of a poor family was removed by disease, his wife and children frequently went into the workhouse, or became beggars. On 8th December 1847 it was resolved that where the head of a family, who had the means to maintain that family, was sent to a fever hospital in the Union, the Relieving Officer on receiving a certificate from the Medical Officer and an application from the family for relief, would recommend 'outdoor relief' on the next Board day. Discharged fever patients were also entitled to relief for a period of up to 4 weeks, if necessary.

Cholera reappeared in Europe in 1847 and the epidemic recurred in Cork before spreading to Limerick and the rest of Munster and part of Connacht in 1849.[20] 503 cases were admitted from 9th March to 16th June. The daily increasing poverty of those seeking admission to the fever wards created a demand for more accommodation, which was met by the new buildings and airing grounds. While the number of admissions was higher in 1845 evidently the quality of the accommodation was important to the Hospital committee. The worth of this well-run, invaluable institution can be gauged by the fact that a relatively low mortality rate was maintained in spite of the moribund condition of some of those admitted. The ratio of deaths to admissions was 1:18 at this period.

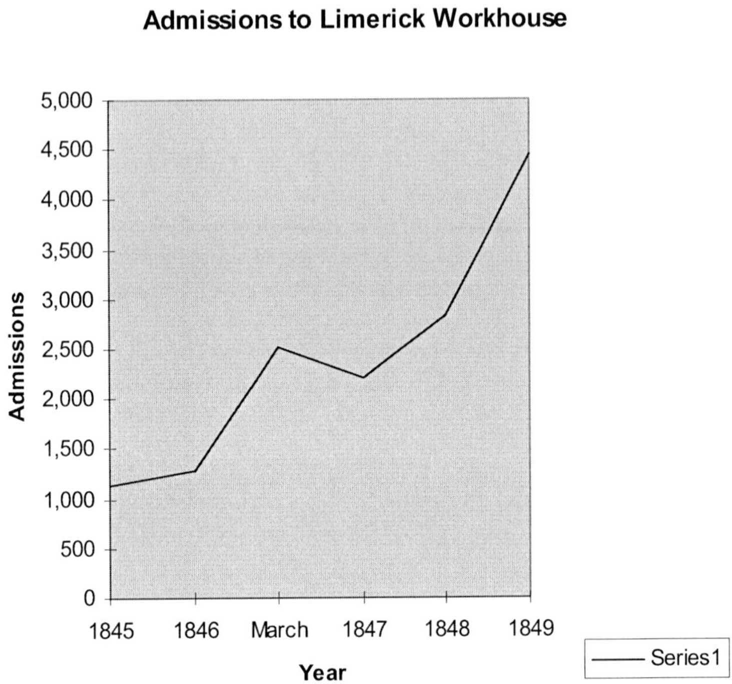

Fig. 15 The pattern of admissions to the workhouse, as opposed to St. John's, gives some idea of the severity of the Famine over time.

At a meeting of the Limerick Union on 20 April 1850 it was resolved that all future cases of fever arising in the Temporary workhouses be removed for treatment to John's Hospital.[21] 520 fever cases were transferred between 29 April and September 1850. At that time the Union workhouse was crowded to the utmost extent, but could not plead contagious disease as an excuse for declining tickets of admission, as these were in St. John's.[22] The agreement with the workhouse was renewed in September 1850.[23]

The hospital was in good working order, capable of meeting all ordinary epidemics at an hour's notice. The Committee, under the chairmanship of the Protestant Bishop, had reason to be pleased with their medical and financial management of the hospital, the relief of the sick poor, and protection of society from the spread of contagious fever. But, by May 1851 Barrington's Hospital was threatening to bring legal action to enforce the Act George 4th, Chap., 58 and 56 whereby 'all fines and penalties imposed be given to the Governors of Barrington's Hospital'.[24] In May 1849 the city magistrates ordered, subject to the opinion of counsel, that petty sessions fines be paid to St. John's Hospital. The Poor Law Commissioners in Dublin, were of the opinion that St. John's had an equitable claim which though it was not supported by the provisions of Irish Poor Law Acts it was clearly in keeping with the spirit.[25] The legal advice was to pay £42 10s 6d, the aggregate of the fines. To add to the financial difficulties, the Guardians cancelled the contract under which fever cases were received from the Auxiliary workhouses of the Union from 30th June, and Mr. Fitzgerald, the Receiver absconded to America with collected rents.[26]

When Barrington's hospital closed as a temporary fever hospital the remaining convalescent cases were transferred to John's Fever Hospital together with bedding. Nearly all the articles were in constant use, during the period of the cholera epidemic. When the matter was discussed at a meeting of the Limerick Union in November 1850, one of those unseemly scenes for which the board was distinguished would have followed but for the intervention of the chairman. At a meeting of the Board of Guardians on 12 December 1850 a motion was put by Mr. Thomas Brown

> That the committee appointed to confer with the Governors of St. John's Hospital, respecting their claim against this union, has not been furnished with the particulars of the clothing, bedding and hospital furniture belonging to the rate payers and which has been removed from Barrington's, to St. John's Hospital without the Guardians' knowledge, I will move on this day fortnight that the resolution adopted this day, ordering payment of a balance purporting to be due to that establishment, shall be rescinded and that the account in question shall be referred to the Finance Committee for examination in accordance with the Board's resolution of the 25th May last, which requires all accounts to be (previous to payment) certified to by a Finance Committee.

By December 1850 St. John's Fever Hospital was advertising private apartments 'with every necessary accommodation and attendance for persons of the better classes who may be attacked with fever and unprovided with suitable accommodation where they reside. The weekly charge £1. 0. 0. being only sufficient to cover expenses'.

It is estimated that out of some 4,000 persons who died in the Limerick Union between 1845-49, 3000 died from cholera.[27] However harrowing life was in the Limerick workhouse, it could not compare with the horrors of the four Clare workhouses in the same period. 'Indeed it may well be that much of the hardship which occurred in the Limerick workhouse derived from the Clare divisions of the union, an overflow of suffering from a county which was devastated in the Famine.'[28] It is estimated that between one and one and a half million people died as a result of the Famine. In the County Limerick town of Hospital there was no official record 'but an oral tradition exists of a much increased death rate in the locality during the later years of the famine', and according to the parish register there were no deaths due to hunger in 1846.[29] Similarly in Boher, in another part of the County, 'many died from famine fever' yet Confirmations took place in Murroe in 1847 which, as Mark Tierney points out, shows that conditions were fairly normal there at the time.[30] The 1851 Census gives deaths in Permanent and Temporary Fever Hospitals between 6th June 1841 to 30 March 1851 in St. John's as 1,960 from fever and 296 from other causes, and 1,318 deaths from fever in temporary hospitals.

Though consumption was by far the most fatal disease affecting the inhabitants of Ireland, the terrible outbreaks of cholera, typhus and typhoid, distracted attention from the ravages of a tuberculosis epidemic.[31] This epidemic, which seems to have begun in the two decades immediately before the Famine, increased in intensity during the second half of the nineteenth century. The great increase in the population, together with the large proportion of young adults, the squalid social conditions and the effects of the Famine, combined to initiate a national epidemic of tuberculosis which lasted for more than a century. Although a decline in tuberculosis set in around 1850, the decline was not sustained and the disease would peak in the late 1890s, and would remain a serious public health problem until the early 1950s.[32]

Improved sanitation and housing, more employment and better wages, together with an increased immunity of survivors of previous epidemics resulted in a steady decline in the numbers admitted to St. John's with fever in the years following the Famine. Lenihan gives the following figures from 1852 - 1864.

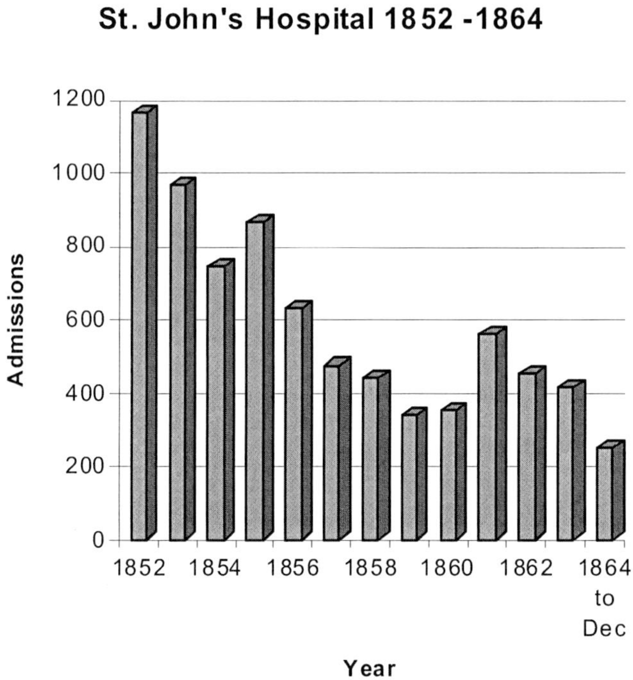

Fig. 16 Limerick Its History and Antiquities

The same general improvement in socio-economic conditions, together with the control (including treatment) of syphilis brought about the decline in morbidity of syphilis in the West from 1860.[33]

The Corporation, as the taxing body of the city, withdrew the annual Grand Jury Grant in 1864. The County Grand Jury continued to support St. John's, which could accommodate nearly 500 patients, admitted people from the county, and because of some bequests, a few city people.[34]

From the late 1860's, towns were forced to appoint Medical Officers of Health, and with other medical staff they taught the science of hygiene and of living organisms. Hygiene became a moral cause, especially in hospitals, which would change from crowded depositories for medical and surgical cases, to well ventilated and supervised wards.[35] Fever, (typhoid and erysipelas) was prevalent in general practice right up to the years between the world wars,[36] but the age of the great epidemics (except the Spanish 'Flu epidemic after World War I), was passing.

In April 1862 Mr Bourk(e), the Poor Law Commission Inspector, reported that an order would be given limiting the number admitted to the workhouse to 2,225. Following a very severe winter, which Mr Carroll, (one of the Guardians of the poor of the Limerick Union), thought was as bad as the famine years 1846-48, the lock hospital had to be enlarged for venereal diseased patients. There were dispensaries for the sick poor in St. John's, St. Michael's, St. Mary's, and St. Munchin's parishes, in the City, and in Caherconlish, Clarina, Coolacasey, Murroe, Annacotty and Bridgetown in the County. Always a champion of the poor of the city Dr. Geary, as Medical Inspector, wrote to the Commissioners on 2 June 1863 regarding the proposal to discontinue the dispensary depot at Nelson Street (St Michael's). He observed that 'the District in question 'contains a population of over 20,000 poor people admitted to gratuitous relief and is divided into four sub-districts'. The effect of closing the depot would impose loss of time on the poorer residents of the sub-district who would have to travel at least one mile to the chief dispensary where additional inconvenience would necessarily arise from the crowded daily attendance there from the three other districts. He requested the Board of Guardians to be good enough to consider their proposition to discontinue the dispensary depot. The committee were unanimous that the amalgamation should go ahead, saying it was more advantageous to the sick poor for many reasons, and will also 'tend to economise the expenditure of the rates'. The Dispensary Committee were further of the opinion that a very small outlay would render the present premises at Barrington's Hospital more than sufficient to accommodate all the sick poor who may apply there for relief.[37] Ill health forced Dr. Geary's retirement at the end of 1863 and the minutes of the Dispensary Committee of the City of Limerick record their 'unanimous opinion of the kind, considerate and efficient manner in which, for several years, he discharged his official duties as Inspector, both as regard the interest of the sick poor as also for his courteous deportment to the members of the Committee'.[38] Dr Geary for his part was for 12 years

> 'glad to have belonged to a group so deeply interested in the welfare of the sick-poor - the zeal and kindly discharge of the duties by the gentlemen of the medical staff - the exemplary efficiency with the blessing of The Medical Charities Act are diffused throughout your largely populated Dispensary District - including as it does about forty thousand persons entitled to claim medical relief under the medical charities act'.[39]

1860-1865 The Limerick Union

On admission to the workhouse, people were classified and segregated by age and gender. The rules required the separation of families. The diet was basic and consisted of bread, stirabout, milk and potatoes, when available. Occasionally there was meat, and when milk was in short supply it was replaced by soup.[40] At a meeting of the Special Committee held on the 7th September 1860, the number of able-bodied Paupers on the books of the Limerick Union at the 1st September was 516. 117 of these were males and 399 were females. 79 males and 175 females were sick.[41]

Inmates were also classified as lunatics, idiots and epileptics and these numbered 50 - 32 females and 18 males. Dr Nugent, Inspector of Lunatic Asylums, generally found the apartments of the lunatic and idiotic classes in the Union to be clean - the rooms well ventilated and the patients, so far as the very limited accommodation of a workhouse allowed, "fairly attended to". However he argued that a Union was a most unsuitable residence for lunatics as they required special treatment and constant supervision as some supposed harmless and tranquil lunatics transferred from the asylum to the workhouse became boisterous and afterwards occasionally showed a violent and dangerous disposition. He also added that it was more economical, and patients had a better hope of recovery in the lunatic asylum, and would cease to be a burden to the public. Nevertheless, only violent lunatics and other inmates requiring restraint were transferred.[42] Clear, writing about female sick poor says:

> "Admission to an asylum was often the penultimate step in a process of deterioration brought on by poorly-paid work or unemployment. Consumption often caused dementia in its final stages, and undiagnosed puerperal fever caused many a woman to be committed to an asylum only to die there two or three days later".[43].

Whatever the reason was for not transferring patients to the lunatic asylum, the Guardians did recommend that in the case of lunatics supposed to be "dangerous" an application be made to the District Lunatic Asylum for their admission before sending them to gaol as was sometimes the case.[44] In December 1863, 17 year old Owen McClusky cut his throat with a razor.[45] There was only one report of an inmate with suicidal tendencies - that was in August 1864.

In 1859, there were on average 432 patients in the workhouse hospital daily and each patient remained in hospital about 65 days. 254 died in that year. Of those, the greater number were incurable - many of them moribund or dying shortly after admission. A large proportion were infants - foundlings - illegitimates - children delicate from birth, and the offspring of diseased/syphilitic parents.[46] By 1837, Clear says, 'female unemployment expressed itself in large numbers of beggars and prostitutes'[47] Patients, on average, remained in a workhouse hospital much longer than in a county or city infirmary - the majority of the cases admitted being of a chronic character. Although a vast number of them were incurable, their diet, medical treatment, relief from pain and other distressing symptoms of their disease, prolonged their existence - in many instances for years. Among other diseases reported in October 1861 were opthalmia among the school children, a great number of whom had to be removed to hospital. At the same time scarlatina appeared in the house, and although widespread in the city and fatal in many cases, out of 30 or 40 cases in the house none died. But even in death there was no rest for them. The Church Yard of Killalee near the City was wholly unfit for further Christian burial and was dangerous to the Public health, according to the Catholic Chaplain of the workhouse. He called on the Guardians as the legally constituted "Burial Board" to apply to his Excellency the Lord Lieutenant for an order in Council to prevent future interments in this church yard. Fr John Quinlan P.P. St John's wanted the church yard closed and a wall built to prevent the desecration of the bodies that were buried there, as he had been informed that the limbs of human beings had been found, by workmen, in the adjacent fields, left by dogs who dragged the corpses from the new made graves.[48] Kileely churchyard also was disrespectful to the dead and dangerous to the Public health and according to Dr Kane the graveyard at Ballynanty was also a problem and needed to be walled in.[49] Eventually, the Board's solicitor, Mr. Joseph Murphy, was granted an injunction to restrain guardians from further internments in the burial ground rented by them from Mr Cullen since 1849[50].

Most of the nursing staff were pauper women lodged in the workhouse. It was difficult to get efficient unpaid nurses to attend the sick, and give them the care and attention that they required. As an incentive to these nurses, the Board of Guardians decided, on the recommendation of the resident medical officer, that they be given an improved diet; i.e. they got more bread and tea or milk. Their duties were unpleasant and difficult, and also dangerous; attending fever, venereal disease, opthalmia, foundlings and lying-in patients. They were expected to attend the sick - remain up at night, if the occasion required it - keep the wards clean - wash the linen of the patients, and the sheets, blankets etc. There were three paid Hospital nurses, and two in the lunatic department. Their rations cost

3s.2d. per week each. The number of unpaid servants was 36, including 2 cooks, a barber and a male infirm ward nurse. The cost of their rations averaged 2s.8d. per week each. The Medical Officer notified the Board that if at any time a sufficient number of nurses could not be procured from the pauper inmates of the House, it would be his duty to call on the Board to provide more paid nurses[51].

Dr Nugent was of the opinion that attendants, who voluntarily devoted themselves to the distressing care of lunatics and epileptics, should receive additional consideration - increased rations. The recommended diet for the hospital nurses and assistants in 1860 was:

1st Class

Breakfast	Dinner	Supper
8oz white bread	10 oz white bread	6 oz white bread
1 pint milk	1 pint of Tea	1 pint milk

8oz meat in place of milk for dinner twice a week

2nd Class was the same as above, with the exception of meat.[52]

There was job rationalisation even in those days. In February 1862, when Mrs Harty tendered her resignation as hospital nurse, it was decided that Miss Geraghty would take charge of her duties. Mrs Hickey would discharge the duties of Miss Geraghty in addition to her own; as Mrs Hickey's former duties had been much lessened there was no need to appoint a successor. Miss Geraghty would have the same salary as Mrs Harty, £12 per year, and keep charge of the female Infirm Ward. Mrs Mack was appointed assistant Female Lock Hospital nurse at £5 with rations.[53] The following year the visiting committee direct that the female lock patients be removed to the new hospital and that the lying-in-patients be transferred to the room occupied at that time by Mrs Mack who would take charge of both departments. In November 1863 her salary was increased to £12 when, having given such satisfaction as nurse, she took charge of the entire female block, Fever, Lock, and Lymph Hospital. Her pay was on a par with Honora Dundon, Assistant Fever Hospital Nurse, and the female lunatic keeper Eliza Enright. Mary Hartney the night nurse got 15/- a quarter more. In 1865 an order was made that she be given 3lbs. of meat weekly in addition to her other rations[54].

The importance of the hospital was increasing every year. The Report of a committee appointed to inquire into the arrangements of the hospital, with the view of promoting the comforts of the sick poor, and to improve their physical and spiritual condition, pointed out the defects in the administration of the hospital. The number of chronic cases has increased and many of the patients when admitted were in a state of great debility and required an 'especial amount of kindly treatment'. The report then becomes critical of the care given to the sick by three paid, and thirty two pauper nurses 'so much of minute and disagreeable attention, as is rarely given by hired nurses, except under the eye of some superintending authority. .... there appears to be an entire absence of moral control over either nurses or patients'[55] .... and even their good diet does not always reach the patients and their daily wants are not satisfactorily provided for. The Sisters of Mercy visited the workhouse to assist the Catholic Chaplain in his duties. The board wanted a central controlling authority to direct the nurses and to make itself respected by the patients - a staff of well-trained nurses and a means of imparting moral and religious instruction. Only trained nurses should be employed, because experience shows, "that the every day management of a large ward (and wards are healthy or unhealthy, mainly, according to the knowledge or ignorance of the nurses in charge of them) is a matter of sufficient importance and difficulty, to require learning by experience and careful inquiry, just as much as any other art". That efficiency could be obtained only by paying high salaries. The board were 'unanimously of opinion, that both in the interest of the poor, and in that of the rate payers, it is expedient to adopt the suggestion made at the last meeting of the board and to invite the Sister of Mercy to take charge of our hospital'.[56]

The Sisters of Mercy were a congregation of women, mainly middle-class, founded in the early nineteenth century, and coinciding with the re-emergence of Catholics into public life. 'Before 1860 visitation of the sick poor was the most prevalent form of nursing care undertaken by nuns. This involved attending the medical and material needs of the poor'[57]. During the cholera epidemic of the 1830s several Sisters of Mercy worked in a public hospital and in 1849 worked in Barrington's and St John's hospitals dealing with an outbreak of fever. By November 1860, out of 1,321 paupers there were 400 in hospital.[58] The Board of Guardians recommended that one sister act as Hospital Matron, with two other Sisters to assist her in the management of the Hospital. Each Sister would receive a salary of £20 per year. However, as early as August 1860, Mr. Monsell, Chairman of the Board of Guardians, 'in a passing way asked if the community would take charge of the Workhouse Hospital in the City;'[59] On 10 November 1860 the Commissioners wrote, quoting extracts from the General Regulations. The question they wanted the Guardians to consider was "whether it is expedient that ladies, whose social position may be regarded as placing them above the ordinary motives which render responsibility practical, should be selected for the performance of the official duties of Nurses and assistants to the Master and Matron of a workhouse". Replying to the Commissioners a week later, it was pointing out that the existing rules were drawn up at a time when hospitals were not expected to form an important part of the workhouse, and did not provide for the skilful and satisfactory administration of the hospital. The Board strongly recommended to the Commissioners that they reconsider their rules and frame a code which would recognise the position and define the duties of a hospital matron. They were warming up for the next meeting of the Board that was attended by 64 members. A tender had been put out for the nursing positions and three applications were received from the Sisters of Mercy. A notice of motion was given that the appointment of the Sisters of Mercy be rescinded. The following week the Commissioners assured the Guardians that 'those Nurses cannot be permitted to possess an authority independent of the authority of the Master and Matron'. The letter went on to state 'that the rules bear the date of the year 1849 when Workhouse Hospitals in Ireland contained nearly twice as many patients as they do at the present, that they were approved by the Lord Lieutenant of that date and cannot be altered without a similar approval'. The rules of the Sisters of Mercy stressed that religious instruction should not be attempted until the ease and comfort of the patient had first been assured[60]. There were only two Protestants in the hospital at this time and though there were conversions to Catholicism, they were few and mostly death-bed. One notable convert was Rosanna Doran, aged 98 who changed her religion from Protestant to Roman Catholic. Nevertheless, notice of motion was given by Mr Cullen that he would move to have a ward in the hospital set apart for Protestant male and female inmates and he would seek leave of the Poor law Commissioners to appoint a Protestant nurse to take care of them. In December 1860 the fear of the Commissioners was that if the Sisters of Mercy were appointed, separate hospitals would be required for Protestant and Catholic inmates, and that Christian Brothers and Sisters of Mercy would be appointed in Poor House schools. They requested the Guardians to readvertise. In a long reply to the Commissioners letter the Guardians state that the real question at issue is whether the poor and dying would be better cared for by mercenary nurses or by Sisters of Mercy - ladies on no salary reporting to a person of lower social order. References to the Emperor Napoleon who reintroduced

Sisters of Charity into hospitals in the Crimea, and to Catholic and Protestant Sisters in the Russian War were made. Their aim was to bring the Limerick union hospital from its present unsatisfactory state up to the same high level which the Vincent Hospital in Dublin and St Elizabeth Hospital in London had already reached. The nursing posts were readvertised and there were only three applicants. It was proposed that Ellen O'Meara be appointed hospital nurse and Ellen Nevill and Anne Curtis be appointed assistant hospital nurses subject to the control and authority of Master and Matron of the Workhouse according to the existing rules. The Sisters first appointed to the hospital were replaced by others at will of the Superior, without reference to the Board of Guardians according to Kelly. The salary was not legally payable to any but those appointed in the prescribed manner,[61] By February the Visitors book contained compliments to the Sisters of Mercy from the Parish Priest of Ennis - the first of many tributes recorded. 'The entry of nuns into local authority hospitals was a very significant gain for Catholic nationalists at a time when the terms 'Catholic' and 'Irish' were becoming increasingly synonymous'.[62] The praise of the Bishops of Clonfert and of Killaloe, recorded in the visitors book, when they visited the hospital in November 1861 is simply Catholic propaganda. They contrast the hospital under the care of the Sisters of Mercy and workhouses elsewhere and

> 'without offering the slightest disparaging remark on the officials in charge of workhouse hospitals generally ..... under no other management than that of Religious could the same advantages to sick paupers be secured as are here the result of Religious superintendence, both as to sanitary treatment and as to the higher and more important matter of the spiritual interests of persons sick and often in immediate danger of death'.

More importantly, the Cork Poor Law Guardians were impressed with the hospitals during their visit in April 1863. Documents relative to the management of the hospitals were sent to Cork and to Ballinasloe Workhouse with the view to enabling them to have Sisters of Mercy admitted to administer to the 'suffering sick poor'. Over 200 inmates received Confirmation in August, so the missionary work of the Sisters, kept pace with the care of the sick.

When Dr. O Flannagan resigned in April 1860 the post was advertised at £75 with rations and an apartment. Moves to improve conditions were afoot in February 1861 by the provision of superannuation or compensation to workhouse staff worn out in such service according to the length and faithfulness of the service rendered. A copy of this resolution, unanimously passed by the Guardians of the South Dublin Union, was received by the Limerick Union. In the same month Dr Brodie was feeling the strain mentally and physically. There were 624 patients in the hospital. Children were suffering from fever and measles and there were about 300 aged and infirm patients. He applied to the Board for some temporary professional assistance but after discussion, it is recorded, he withdrew his application. Fever in the city was severe and likely to continue for some time and the Inspector, Mr Bourk, recommended that Dr Brodie be given assistance should he ask again. In December 1861 Dr. P.H. Keon moved to Drumshambo dispensary. An advertisement for his successor offered £100 with rations and an apartment - a 33.3% increase in salary. In February 1862, Mr Hall, one of the Guardians, gave notice of a motion to have Dr. Brodie's salary increased to £120 a year, as his duties had increased much and that sum being the salary he enjoyed when he undertook the responsible duties of sole visiting officer of the house. In June 1864 Lord Clarina championed the cause of Dr. Brodie whom he said received inadequate remuneration for his services as principal and responsible Medical Officer of the workhouse, - a vast general infirmary containing between 700 - 800 sick. The additional duties were imposed on him as a consequence of the withdrawal of the city grand jury grant for the support of the Fever hospital and city infirmary. A large fever hospital was by this time attached to the workhouse. In addition, recent legislation on Births, Marriages and Deaths became Dr Brodie's responsibility also. He was offered an increase in salary of £50 a year. This enraged James Ryan one of the Guardians who tried to have the increase rescinded. In a blistering attack on Dr. Brodie, he claimed that influence was brought to bear and it was useless to oppose. He also stated that Mr Carroll (who had a son a doctor) had proposed an amendment which he subsequently withdrew; that Dr Brodie attended the workhouse for two hours daily; as Medical Officer of the Clarina dispensary he received £100, totaling '£220 out of the rates of the Limerick Union - together with the practice of so able and popular a man among his friends ought be ample for a man disencumbered as he is - having no want but the want of more'.[63] Dr Brodie was in charge of the female departments of the infirmary and fever hospital and the male departments were in Dr O'Sullivan's charge. These institutions were a matter for congratulations from Dr Parker and the visiting Committee in April 1864, when new lunatic wards and the fever hospital were said to provide ample accommodation. In November, the order of October 1862 was replaced and it became necessary for the applicant to have a Diploma in Surgery and a Midwifery Certificate to compete for an appointment as workhouse dispensary Medical Officer.

Dr O Sullivan, the resident Medical Officer of the house had a more difficult time, being the subject, together with Miss Geraghty, of a long scurrilous letter sent to the Board of Guardians. It complained of Miss Geraghty's upgrading to Matron 'pro tem' saying bad conduct had been rewarded when it should have been punished. It alleged that a good many in the house thought that Miss Geraghty and Dr O'Sullivan were married and invited the Gentlemen of the Board to draw their own conclusions. The letter was signed "an official". Both of the accused denied the allegations and requested that a sworn enquiry be held, which the Guardians requested the Commissioners to do. The enquiry revealed that the letter was written by the Rev Mr. Slattery and the united testimony of the workhouse staff was that there was nothing improper in their conduct. It thought it remarkable that Mr Slattery never protested or cautioned either of the parties concerned and never consulted the chaplain - on whose behalf he was acting. The Guardians were requested to consider whether it was desirable that Slattery continue to assist the Roman Catholic Chaplain of the workhouse. Slattery himself was unrepentant except to say that he should have signed the letter. His actions are indefensible but in an institution which kept husbands and wives apart, a less than business-like relationship between officers of the workhouse may have caused more anguish in the inmates. He claimed his object was to promote the order, discipline and morality of the house.

The Board of Guardians had many problems to contend with. The record for 31 March 1860 shows that no one was relieved out of the workhouse, at that date. The weekly average for maintenance of paupers was 2s.1d. per head. The hospital building was constantly under alteration due to increased numbers of different classes of patients or the effects of the weather. In February 1861 there was insufficient room for the number of females in the lunatic department. The following month the windows of the hospital were admitting wind and rain during inclement weather, causing very great inconvenience and even danger to the patients. The roof of the fever hospital needed repairs having sustained considerable damage in a storm[64].

The visiting committee in 1862 decided that all pauper males over 15 years should break stones as a test. The following year a Resolution passed that all healthy men over 15 years of age registered in the workhouse, be employed in stone breaking, including the men in the shoemaker's shop, and that the schoolboys alone be engaged by the officers of the house as clerks and messengers. The record shows that men laboured for 8 hours a day while schoolboys worked 5 hours in the field and 3 in the classroom.

When a contractor went before the board saying the work could not go on if he lost the help of labourers, it was recommended that the able-bodied men who were discharged be readmitted for a fortnight to help the mason finish on time, there being no other able bodied men at present to take their place.[65]

Nothing was manufactured in the workhouse, and no farm attached to it. The only produce grown were vegetables and the sum credited for these was £39.17.6 in March and £29.19.0 in September. No potatoes were planted on the workhouse site that autumn. It was perhaps just as well. A circular received from the Commissioners in October regarding the state of the potato crop stated that a considerable portion was unfit for human consumption, and they pointed out the necessity of being prepared for the possible increase in the number of applicants for relief. This was a recurring problem over the years.[66]

Milk was in short supply in winter. The large quantity bought by the Union caused the price in the milk market to rise, creating more problems for the poor of the city. As a consequence, the Doctor was asked by the Board of Guardians to revise the diet of the inmates. Coffee and soup were given in place of some milk. The bread was frequently reported as not satisfactory and the poor of the house suffered as a result. The stirabout was not good in November 1863 and ordered to be made of 2/3 Indian corn and 1/3 oatmeal. In December that year a riot broke out. Nineteen of the men refused their stirabout. One named Costelloe struck wardmaster Hickey. They then went to the Master's parlour and attacking his room in a violent manner, demanded another breakfast. This was refused as the Master considered the one served was good. They then took over the dining hall and would not leave. The Master sent for the police and a large force arrived from Thomondgate and Cahirdavin. George Hayes, the porter, was passing down the hall when William Lawrence made a thrust at him with a knife. Fortunately, the knife bent and merely cut through his clothes. John Gavin, also attacked Hayes and subsequently kicked him in the face. While this was going on the able-bodied women were in the yard shouting and throwing stones at the windows of the dining hall. The police dispersed them and arrested some of the most violent together with the male ringleaders. Those convicted got prison sentences, all with hard labour. Lawrence was sentenced to penal servitude for life and Gavin got one year with hard labour[67].

The Union was in debt - owing the sum of £1,523 to the Bank, and the rates, which supported the workhouse, were not collected in full and in a nine month period in 1861 expenditure exceeded the estimate by about

£1,500. The Bank wanted repayment of the loan. In February 1862 the workhouse could accommodate 2058 inmates. In April the debt was £4,000 and the amount of irrecoverable rates was £500. There was a large increase in the number of aged and infirm inmates and the number of women and children deserted by their husbands and parents respectively. In August 1863 another loan of £1,000 was applied for to the National Bank, at a rate of 5% interest, to pay the expense of erection and completion of the new hospital. A request was made that the overdraft of £4,500 be allowed to remain out until 1st November, as due to the distressed state of the ratepayers the amount could not be collected until after the harvest. It was not until February 1864 that Mr Bourk, the Inspector, could claim that the financial condition of the union had improved.

Emigration from the workhouse might have improved the financial position of the union but it wasn't approved of generally. One fantastic scheme suggested by Mrs Villiers Boyd[68] proposed sailing to Queensland, where she hoped to obtain a Government grant of 5,000 acres of land with the view to establishing an industrial school to train children to cultivate cotton and silk. She asked the Board to consider paying the passages of the number of boys in the workhouse aged from 7 to 14, promising to give the children every opportunity of developing their intellectual powers, and bringing each child up in the professed Religion of his parents. It was turned down.

In May 1862 the Commissioners forwarded information, issued by the Government Emigration Office in Quebec, for assistance to would-be emigrants. Inmates who had relatives in the colonies and who sent some money to them were assisted to emigrate. These were few and infrequent. The only large-scale emigration in the period 1860 - 65 happened in October 1864 when thirty young women left the workhouse, in charge of the removing office to Liverpool for Quebec - 'the last steamer to sail up the St. Lawrence' [presumably before the river froze over for the Winter months].

A report from the Secretary of the National Education in July 1860 said that the children (a ray of hope in a very bleak house) appeared reasonably clean and healthy and that the pupils exhibited a considerable amount of quickness and intelligence[69]. By March 1862 the Secretary was testing the knowledge of the boys of third (highest) class on the basic subjects required for the study of navigation. Limerick was, at that time, the only workhouse in Ireland in which this branch of study was introduced. It was the brainchild of the Rev. Dean Keating, of Kilfenora. Permission was granted by the Commissioners in August 1861 to allow Mr Patrick Murray, the teacher of the Limerick Maritime School, to attend for three days a week, to give lessons on navigation. It was hoped to give the boys an advantage over the majority of those applying for seafaring jobs and to put promotion prospects within their grasp once employed. The Guardians were legally empowered to supply apprentices to the sea service alone, and the course in navigation did not interfere with any trade. The class consisted of fourteen boys whose ages ranged from nine to fourteen years. Mr Murray commenced teaching geometry, algebra, decimal fractions and mathematical geography. By 30th August 1862 they were being examined by the District Inspector, in these subjects, together with the elements of trigonometry and navigation. They had been instructed in four books of Euclid. Six of the boys were able to demonstrate most of the propositions contained in the course, and others, nearly all the propositions of the first book. It was a remarkable achievement. Six were fully qualified for apprenticeship to the merchant navy. Female children spent one hour daily devoted to needlework - making and mending their own clothes; knitting and embroidery.[70]

In early August, John Barron (17) and Lawrence Harman (15) were, at their own request, apprenticed to the sea service for four years. Their employer was a Mr Hodgson of Northumberland, who agreed to pay £5 for the first year; £6 for the second; £7 for the third and £8 for the fourth year. An additional £2 would be paid with 12/- in lieu of washing, on the faithful completion of the entire service. By May of 1863 the boys had come home to the Limerick Union and the Board directed the Clerk to write to the ship's master to ask if he would take them back.[71]

The visiting committee found the infant school was anything but satisfactory - the clothing of the children entirely neglected and the windows completely broken by the children for want of proper supervision. A couple of months later the District Inspector suggests that Miss Roberts the infant class teacher be allowed 'to attend occasionally at one of the infant schools in the city either in the model or that under the direction of the Sisters of Mercy and St Mary's Convent in order that she may witness the mode of teaching and become acquainted with the organization and general management'.[72]

1887-1890 St. John's Hospital

St. John's was a large hospital, with convalescent wards, and almost three acres of land adjoining. It had few, sometimes no patients and funds were low.

At a meeting in January 1887 management decided to put the two nurses on half pay until further notice. The committee reserved the right to reverse this decision, in order to keep the hospital open in the event of any epidemic breaking out in the city. The staff's coal allowance was also reduced to one ton per annum. The secretary's salary was reduced to £5. per annum. Instead of paying the hospital physician Dr. Gelston a fixed yearly sum, the committee decided that he should be paid a piece rate of 2 guineas per consultation, up to a maximum of £20 in any one year.[73] Dr. Gelston retired from the Staff soon afterwards, the last physician to work in the old St. John's Fever and Lock Hospital.[74]

By November 1887, there was an accession of new governors including the Catholic Bishop of Limerick, Dr. Edward O'Dwyer who joined the Governing Body with a view to resuscitating the hospital through tapping new sources of funding and gifts. The Bishop became chairman of the new Board and management of St. John's Fever Hospital which now passed into Catholic control.

By January 1888 it was apparent that the new Governors proposed making considerable alterations and improvements in the construction of the hospital with a view to having trained nursing nuns in residence and making it more useful for the general public. Under such circumstances they did not think it advisable to place the dividends in a fund to be used only in case of an outbreak of fever in the city. The Catholic Church, like the other Churches, had as its aims the evangelisation and civilisation of the poor. Most of the Catholics working in schools, hospitals and other institutions, particularly from the 1840s, were women religious.[75] Most nursing nuns worked for the local authority in workhouse hospitals and city infirmaries. On 1st September 1888 the committee received a £1,000 donation from Count Moore, a wealthy patron, for the establishment of the sisters of the Little Company of Mary in the city, and for the necessary fitting up of their living quarters in the hospital.

When Moore visited Rome in 1885, his wife fell dangerously ill and was nursed back to health by sisters of the Little Company of Mary. Both wished to bring the nursing order to Ireland and they approached Dr. O'Dwyer, Bishop of Limerick.[76] O'Dwyer hoped that the sisters would take charge of a public hospital, the long disused St. John's Hospital which he was "practically in possession of"[77] in November 1887. He wanted to meet the Mother Superior in Limerick to discuss the requisite structural changes to the building. The first work of the sisters was the removal and burial of infectious articles of bedding, left over from the fever epidemics. The hospital reopened on 10 October 1888.[78]

A paid nurse was considered as an ignorant and unskilled servant and no respectable person would do that work, until Florence Nightingale raised it to the status of a profession, with her outstanding work at Scutari and in the Crimea in 1850s.[79] Her system improved nursing discipline and hospital organization. The Little Company of Mary was the first Catholic Religious congregation founded in England since the Reformation for the purpose of nursing the sick. Their founder, Mother Mary Potter, was anxious that her companions became skillful nurses in their work of caring for the sick and dying.[80] In 1897 Dr. Mulcahy, a Limerick general practitioner, lectured the sisters in anatomy and physiology and set examinations for them, but they were not allowed to nurse maternity cases, to undertake night duty, or to nurse male patients: 'as modesty must never be wounded, nor is it necessary that it should be; a suitable person will be provided by the Mother Superior to render these services'. These restrictions must have caused them to be compared unfavourably with lay nurses.[81]'

Life for the sisters was made extremely difficult in those early days by the Catholic authority in Limerick.

> When the Company arrived in Limerick in 1888 O'Dwyer was displeased that he had not been given sufficient notice (the sisters were assured that he had), and when he taxed Mother Veronica for this, 'she being I dare say new to responsibility and not knowing the character of the bishop said that if his Lordship did not choose to have them other bishops would gladly welcome them to their dioceses'. The Sisters of Mercy intervened and got Mother Veronica to apologise to O'Dwyer, and so the community's trouble with the bishop 'ended amicable for the time being in any case', as the annals ominously state.[82]

The permanent staff of sisters for hospital duty was never to be less than four, and each would receive £25 a year.[83] Their accommodation was extremely damp and it was agreed, in February 1889, to have partitions put up between their rooms and the passage. When one of the sisters died, an application was made to the management committee for payment of a coffin. It was proposed by the chairman, the Rev. J. O'Shea, and unanimously agreed that they could not see their way to accede to the request![84] Money might not be forthcoming but there was plenty of direction. Reverend Mother was instructed that a requisition must be sent to the treasurer for any articles necessary for the hospital, as the management committee would not be responsible for goods supplied without their sanction.[85] Between 1 May 1888 - 11 July 1890 222 patients were treated.

Notes

[1] The Limerick Chronicle 1826. Gearóid Ó Tuathaigh, Ireland Before the Famine 1798-1848, (Dublin 1991). (hereafter Ó Tuathaigh, Ireland Before the Famine). In the North, the demand for cotton ceased and about 10,000 Belfast weavers were out of work, but the industry recovered when an investment in new machines for spinning linen was made.
[2] Adam Smith's 'Wealth of Nations', advocating the doctrine of Laissez-faire, appeared in 1776.
[3] Ó Tuathaigh, Ireland Before the Famine pp 118-119, p 122, p 129
[4] Porter, Cambridge Illustrated History of Medicine, p 46.
[5] Ó Tuathaigh, Ireland Before the Famine, pp 134-7.
[6] J.C. Beckett, A Short History of Ireland, (London 1971) p 108.
[7] George O'Brien, The Economic History of Ireland from the Union to the Famine, (New Jersey 1972) pp 235-6.
[8] Minute Book Barrington's Hospital. O'Brien State Intervention and the Medical Relief. p 205. Under the Poor Law Amendment Act (1843) workhouses were empowered to build fever hospitals when necessary.
[9] Dr. Gelston, a Limerick doctor
[10] M. F. O'Sullivan, A history of Hospital and its environs, (Tipperary 1995), p 51. hereafter O'Sullivan, A history of Hospital and its environs.
[11] The Limerick Chronicle 13 January, 1847
[12] British Parliamentary Papers, Famine (Ireland), Vol. 7. 1847 p 66. Letter dated February 2, 1847 from Dr. Gelston to Commissary-General Hewetson on 'the diminution of disease in this locality'.
[13] Barrington's Hospital Archive.
[14] A balance of £665 7s 3d was on hand on 6th January 1845, and an amount of £507 13s 0d was collected in the City during the Autumn and Winter, and a £100 bequest of the late Earl of Limerick. St. John's Hospital Archive
[15] St. John's Hospital Archive 1st August 1848.
[16] Dr. William J. Geary J.P. had an active interest in local politics and was Mayor of Limerick in 1844 when Mathew Bridge was built. Lenihan, Limerick Its History and Antiquities, p 346. In 1826 he was Treasurer of the Sick Poor Fund and was appointed secretary to the Limerick Mechanics Institute. A great debt of gratitude was owed to Dr. Wm. Geary and his father before him who gave such devoted service to the sick and poor people of Limerick. Wm. Geary, a Governor for life of St. John's, was appointed medical inspector at the end of 1851.
[17] Ciarán Ó Murchadha, 'Limerick Union Workhouse During the Great famine' Old Limerick Journal, Famine Edition No. 32, Winter 1995.
[18] Chris O'Mahony The Poor Law Comes to Limerick', The Old Limerick Journal No. 6, 1980.
[19] Dom Mark Tierney, OSB, Murroe and Boher, the history of an Irish county parish, (Dublin 1966) (hereafter Tierney Morroe and Boher) p 127.
[20] Cork Fever Hospital medical report. According to the report a donation of £50 was received from the Queen. British Parliamentary Papers Famine (Ireland) 8

Appendix B. No. 6 Summary of Returns gives the number of Cholera cases between 26th February 1849 and 7 September 1849 for Limerick as 1,500 and Cholera deaths as 746. On p 440 the population of Limerick is given as 65,296.

[21] Extract from minutes of Limerick Union - 20 April 1850. Ciarán Ó Murchadha For most of the famine period, the two main auxiliaries were at Boherbuoy and Mount Kenneth. Other buildings in William Street (March, 1849) and Clare Street (December, 1849) were rented out for short periods and soon closed.

[22] Covering letter dated 29 August 1850.

[23] Minutes of Board of Guardians Limerick Union, 10 September 1850

[24] Mark Tierney, 'The Origins and Early Years of Barrington's Hospital' in The Old Limerick Journal, November 24, 1988, p 38.

[25] Letter 14 September 1850

[26] Letter J. Boyse upper Mallow Street 18 December 1850. Joseph Murphy, Dublin acting for the Charities under Miss Whites will wrote in 1851 to Dr. W.J. Geary about the loss of money. The deficiency was created by not requiring the receiver, to account regularly, and by not appointing a new one when Fitzgerald left the country.

[27] Tierney, Murroe and Boher p 127.

[28] Ciarán Ó Murchadha 'Limerick Union Workhouse During the Great famine' in The Old Limerick Journal Famine Edition. British Parliamentary Papers 1851 Census p 648 The population of Limerick city increased by 10.45% (5,057) between 1841 and 1851. Those born in adjoining counties numbered 9,978, and born in Clare 7,375. No figures are available for those who emigrated.

[29] M. F. O'Sullivan, A history of Hospital and its environs, p 51.

[30] Mark Tierney Old Limerick Journal Famine Edition No. 32, Winter 1995.

[31] The Report of the Commissioners for the 1841 Census.

[32] James Deeny, Tuberculosis in Ireland p 24

[33] King and Nicol, Venereal Diseases p 3

[34] Lenihan, Limerick Its History and Antiquities, pp. 370-371.

[35] Porter, Cambridge History of Medicine p 321

[36] Porter, Cambridge History of Medicine p 150

[37] Minute book of the Limerick Union 1863

[38] Ibid.

[39] Ibid.

[40] Minute books of the Limerick Union 1860

[41] Minute books of the Limerick Union 8 September 1860

[42] Minute books of the Limerick Union 1860

[43] Caitriona Clear, Nuns in Nineteenth Century Ireland, Dublin 1987, p.12.

[44] Minute books of the Limerick Union 19 November 1864

[45] Minute books of the Limerick Union 1864

[46] Minute books of the Limerick Union 1860

[47] C. Clear, Nuns in Nineteenth Century Ireland p.15

[48] Minute books of the Limerick Union August 1860

[49] Minute books of the Limerick Union 1861and 1864.

[50] Minute books of the Limerick Union 1865
[51] Minute books of the Limerick Union
[52] Minute books of the Limerick Union July 1860
[53] Minute book of the Limerick Union 1862
[54] Minute books of the Limerick Union 1865
[55] Minute books of the Limerick Union 1860
[56] Ibid.
[57] C. Clear, Nuns in Nineteenth-Century Ireland p.126.
[58] Minute books of the Limerick Union 3 November 1860
[59] Convent of Our Lady of Mercy, St Mary's Limerick 1838-1939 p.59.
[60] C. Clear, Nuns in Nineteenth-Century Ireland, p.126.
[61] Sr Patricia Kelly, From Workhouse to Hospital The Role of the Irish Workhouse in Medical Relief to 1921, UCG 1972, p.138.
[62] C Clear, Nuns in Nineteenth-Century Ireland, p.132
[63] Minute books of the Limerick Union
[64] Minute books of the Limerick Union 1861
[65] Minute books of the Limerick Union December 1863
[66] Minute books of the Limerick Union
[67] Minute books of the Limerick Union 1863
[67] Minute books of the Limerick Union 1863
[68] Minute books of the Limerick Union December 1863
[69] Minute books of the Limerick Union July 1860
[70] Minute books of the Limerick Union March 1862
[71] Minute books of the Limerick Union 1863
[72] Minute books of the Limerick Union 1864
[73] St. John's Hospital Archive. In March 1861 minute book of the Limerick Union records 'There is as much trouble about the appointment of Dr Gelston in a dispensary who is very well qualified but not quite 23 yrs of age as required by regulation'.
[74] J F Devane, MD, A History of St. John's Hospital Limerick, p 31
[75] Caitriona Clear Nuns in Nineteenth Century Ireland (Dublin 1987), p xvi (hereafter Clear Nuns in Nineteenth Century Ireland).
[76] Patick Dougherty, Mother Mary Potter, Foundress of the Little Company of Mary (1847-1913) (London 1961), (hereafter Dougherty, Mother Mary Potter), pp 176-7 Archbishop Croke of Cashel was first approached but turned the idea down. O'Dwyer of the neighbouring diocese of Limerick was then consulted.
[77] St. John's Hospital Archive
[78] Dougherty, Mother Mary Potter, pp.177-9
[79] Dougherty, Mother Mary Potter, pp.230-1. See also Cambridge History of Medicine.
[80] Dougherty, Mother Mary Potter, p 232.
[81] Clear, Nuns in Nineteenth Century Ireland, p.127, 129
[82] Clear, Nuns in Nineteenth Century Ireland, p 63
[83] St. John's Hospital Minutes of meeting dated 18 December 1888

[84] St. John's Hospital Minutes of meeting dated 12 December 1890.
[85] St. John's Hospital Minutes of meeting dated 5 April 1889

CHAPTER SIX

CONCLUSION

This study deals to a large extent with the 1820s, and to a lesser extent with the 1840s a period when admissions to St. John's hospital peaked. However, admissions in the 1820s were numerous enough to form a significant statistical base.

The eighteenth century brought several major epidemics. During the 1741 famine smallpox, dysentery, typhus and relapsing fever became epidemical. From 1771–1772, when food was again scarce, there was a marked increase of fever. In the eighteenth and nineteenth centuries epidemics of fever were frequent and no institutional care was available anywhere in the British Empire, prior to the setting up of St. John's Hospital in 1780. The poor suffered and died in their homes from typhus, typhoid, and relapsing fever, dysentery, tuberculosis, smallpox and various other diseases. They were frequently hungry, and their streets, lanes and homes were filthy. St. John's hospital attempted to prevent the spread of fever by isolating fever patients. In the beginning, a ward was set aside for venereally diseased women, but the hospital admitted infected males and children also. Whenever fever became epidemical, venereally diseased patients were reluctantly discharged from St. John's in order to provide more accommodation for fever patients. In addition, large numbers of the sick poor received advice and medicine from the hospital and doctors occasionally visited them in their homes.

Typhoid was endemic in the city between 1786-87 and 1791-92 when food prices were high and people starved. Following the rebellion of 1798, bad weather in 1799 caused a crop failure, and yet another epidemic ensued. The conditions of the poor in the principal towns in Ireland in the years 1799-1802 were miserable. In order to buy food for the day, the poor pawned their clothes, thereby exposing themselves to cold, increasing filth and having to crowd together for warmth. St. John's admissions increased to almost double that of any year since its foundation. This was a dangerous and frequently fatal fever yet mortality in St. John's was 6 per cent or less during this epidemic. The site of the city was not unhealthy but malnourishment and insanitary living conditions, together with the presence of soldiers, who were frequently quartered on families and spread disease, ensured that misery was ever present. The old town decayed and the poverty of those who remained there grew.

The next big epidemic occurred between 1817-1819 when typhus ravaged Ireland. In these years patients were admitted to the hospital who had not eaten for days. Numbers were greater than the hospital could hold and a charitable benefactor provided a temporary hospital from January 1818. This epidemic was worse than the previous one because the end of the Napoleonic wars, together with a rising population and agricultural depression brought mass unemployment. Merchants and manufacturers became bankrupts. Many people became destitute and mendicant. Mortality was highest in 1818 at over 8 per cent, mainly from dysentery and the twenty to thirty age group were most vulnerable. In the following year mortality fell to less than 3 per cent. St. John's had learnt some valuable lessons which would explain its success in treating fever patients. First, on admission of patients to hospital, it was normal practice to cut their hair short or even shave their heads. Patients were bathed and dressed in clean bed clothes, and beds were changed at least once daily. This routine hygienic practice would have kept contagion to a minimum and aided recovery. Secondly, Dr. John Geary would appear to have been a good diagnostician and had no difficulty in telling typhus from typhoid fever, as early as 1820[1]. Thirdly, patients were given nourishing food and their 'cures' became less aggressive.

The Register of patients at St. John's Hospital between 1821 and 1826 recorded details of more than 10,000 patients, the vast majority were labourers and their dependents and were admitted with fever. Almost one half of all admissions were aged eleven to twenty. The twenty to thirty age group comprised just a quarter of those admitted. Most admissions took place during the 'hunger months' of June, July, and August, between the end of the old season's potato crop and the beginning of the new crop. Despite the increasing precautions taken against contagion, poverty increased the incidence of fever, and admissions to St. John's grew rapidly in this period. The harvest failed again in 1822, and the consequences are well documented. The register of admissions to St. John's, together with newspaper reports covering the period 1825-1826, provide statistical information to validate anecdotal evidence of this epidemic. The situation worsened in 1826 when some patients were admitted to St. John's, who were dying of starvation. Relapses were frequent. Fever cases were numerous in various parts of the city, and the hospital was crowded. Patients lay on the floor between the beds, and the hospital needed funds to meet its increased expenditure. The amount of time a patient spent in hospital varied. In general, venereal patients stayed longer than fever patients, but for either of them it could be a long wait for death. The staff of the hospital, particularly the nurses (extraordinary women doing very difficult and dangerous work), suffered from, and in some cases died of fever. Those who survived the frequent epidemics increased their immunity.

The streets of Limerick in 1825 were crowded nightly with prostitutes. Many had venereal disease, especially mendicants, but most suffered from fever. Other admissions included young poor scholars. Ship-board fever was one of the most deadly and concentrated forms of typhus and the hospital provided an invaluable service in preventing its spread by admitting sailors with fever.

The Sick Poor Fund was set up to relieve convalescent patients discharged from the fever hospital by distributing nourishing food, and large amounts of straw. It maintained 844 people per week; the daily average 62 people at a cost of three-half-pence each. The ratio of deaths to admissions fell from an average 1 in 17.83 to an average 1 in 19.52 between 1822-1826. The sustained improvement in treatment (even in the absence of an accurate knowledge of the real causes of fever) is evidenced by reductions in the ratio of deaths to admissions.

When the Cholera epidemic of 1832 arrived in Limerick St. John's was fitted out in the belief that it would accommodate any number of cases that might arise. Dr. William Geary, son of Dr. John Geary was appointed Inspector. The disease became virulent from 26th May when several people died of Cholera, spreading terror and dismay throughout the city. Barrington's opened on 12th June to receive Cholera patients, and the Nunnery, the Christian Brothers School and Rose Tavern were converted into temporary hospitals. On average four people died in their homes to every one person who died in hospital. The death rate reached 154 per week by the end of June. The epidemic was of short duration, about two month, but of the 2,602 cases of Cholera admitted to hospitals, 953 died.

The outbreak of famine fever in Limerick City in 1845 saw St. John's Hospital coping with more than 5,000 fever-ridden patients, while as many more could not be admitted due to lack of accommodation. The 1845 intake was almost double that of Dublin's Cork Street, yet the average rate of mortality was lower in St. John's at 6.38 per cent, due, perhaps, to better care or nourishment, or both. Admissions to St. John's fell to 2,204 during

1846. These figures suggest an improvement in 'black' 47, which, if true, would contradict the trends countrywide and in the famine-stricken hinterland. Moreover, animals slaughtered in the city for export would have provided a good deal of offal, with which the poor could make nourishing soups and meat dishes. Public works gave some employment for a time, yet the streets swarmed with country paupers. Some relief was given by the Society of Friends who operated soup kitchens. Auxiliary workhouses opened in the Summer of 1847 to take the excess from the main Workhouse where mortality was very high. Lock patients were sent to St. John's from the workhouse. Income was down in 1847, admissions increased by more than a third to 3,525, and expenditure was up by almost 100 per cent. Only the increased contributions from the County and City Grand Juries prevented closure of St. John's.

Cholera reappeared in Limerick in 1849, and 503 cases were admitted to St. John's between 9th March to 16th June. In spite of the moribund condition of some of those admitted, a relatively low mortality rate of 7.75 per cent, (compared to the return of the Board of Health of 38.44 per cent) was maintained. When the temporary fever hospitals closed, fever cases were transferred for treatment to St. John's Fever Hospital. Most of the city poor were migrants from the countryside. Of the estimated 3000 people who died of cholera in the Limerick Union between 1845-1849, it would appear that most came from the Clare divisions of the union, where conditions were so much worse. The 1851 Census gives deaths between 1841-1851 in St. John's as 1,960 from fever and 296 from other causes, and 1,318 deaths from fever in temporary hospitals. Voluntary and ad hoc responses to epidemics worked in the various crises but were patently inadequate to cope with fevers in the Great Famine.

Microbial pathogens were discovered to be the prime source of disease, in the late nineteenth-century. With more precise categorization and causation established by Pasteur and Koch, the generic 'fever' would disappear.

---

[1] Geary, A Historical and Medical Report p.24, Barker and Cheyne An account of the fever lately epidemical p.20.

BIBLIOGRAPHY

Microfilm of St. John's Hospital Archive material, Limerick Regional Archives.

St. John's Hospital Archive. Papers did not include the hospital register for 1820s.

Minute Book, Barrington's Hospital 25 November 1846, Glenstal Abbey.

Historical Records of the Existence and Progress of Cholera in the City of Limerick, During the Months of May and June, 1832. Limerick, 1832.

British Parliamentary Papers

1821 Census, H.C. 1823.

1831 Census.

Reports of the Commissioners appointed to take the Census of Ireland for the year 1841, Dublin 1843, p xxiv. Report upon the Tables of Deaths p ii.

Correspondence relating to the measures adopted for the relief of distress in Ireland Board of Works Series Famine (Ireland) 7. 1847.

Reports from the Relief Commissioners and other papers on Famine Relief in Ireland 1846-53. Famine (Ireland) 8, pp.xix-xx.

1851 Census Ireland; Part vi, General Report, Vol. 14, Census of parishes Vol. 12.

The Limerick Chronicle 1825

—. 1826

—. 1847

Aalen, F.H.A., Whelan, Kevin, and Stout, Matthew (eds.), Atlas of the Irish Rural Landscape, Cork 1997.

Barker, F. and Cheyne, J. An account of the rise, progress and decline of the fever lately epidemical in Ireland together with communications from physicians in the provinces and various official documents Vol. I Dublin 1821

Beckett, J.C. A Short History of Ireland, Fourth edition London 1971

Bryder, Linda, Below the Magic Mountain, a social history of tuberculosis in twentieth century Britain, Oxford 1988.

Clear, Caitriona Nuns in Nineteenth Century Ireland, Dublin 1987.

Clarkson, L.A. and Crawford, E. M., ‘Life after Death: Widows in Carrick-on-Suir, 1799’. In Margaret MacCurtain and Mary O’Dowd, (eds.). Women in Early Modern Ireland, Edinburgh 1991

Cullen, L.M. An Economic History of Ireland since 1660, London 1978.

Curtis, Edmund, A History of Ireland, London 1968.

Deeny, James M.D. Tuberculosis in Ireland - Report of the National Tuberculosis Survey (1950-53) n.p.1954.

Devane, J. F. M.D., F.R.C.S.I. A History of St John’s Hospital Limerick. 1970.

Dickson, David, Arctic Ireland, Belfast 1998.

Dougherty, Patick, Mother Mary Potter, Foundress of the Little Company of Mary (1847-1913) London 1961.

Duffy, Seán, (General Editor) Atlas of Irish History, Dublin 1997.

Farmar, Tony, (ed.) The end of an epidemic, selected essays in Irish public health 1935-1965 by James Deeny, Dublin 1995.

Ferrar, John, The History of Limerick, Limerick 1787.

Geary, John M.D. A Historical and Medical Report of the Limerick Fever and Lock Hospitals, Limerick 1820.

Granshaw, Lindsay. The rise of the modern hospital in Britain. In Andrew Wear (ed.). Medicine in Society, Historical Essays. Cambridge, 1993.

Griffin, Daniel M.D. An Enquiry into the Mortality occurring among the Poor of the City of Limerick. Quarterly Journal of the Statistical Society of London, 1841 Vol. iii, Part iv.

Gwynn, A. and Hadcock, RN, Medieval Religious Houses Ireland, London 1970.

Hennessy, M.A., C.E., A Scheme for a water supply to the city of Limerick published by J.F. O’Gorman, Limerick 1879.

Hill, Judith The Building of Limerick, Cork 1991.

Jones, Greta, and Malcolm, Elizabeth (eds.) Medicine, Disease and the State in Ireland, 1650-1940 Cork 1999. Gerard O’Brien, State Intervention and the Medical Relief of the Irish Poor, 1787-1850, Crawford, E. Margaret, Typhus in Nineteenth-Century Ireland.

Joyce, Gerry, Limerick City Street Names Limerick Corporation, 1995.

Kavanagh, Bernard, MD, Sanitary State of Limerick - a letter addressed to the Right Worshipful Robert McMahon, J.P., Mayor of Limerick and to the members of the Town Council Limerick 1863.

Kemmy, Jim, The Limerick Anthology, Dublin 1996.

—. The Limerick Compendium, Dublin 1997.

King, Ambrose and Nicol, Claude, Venereal Diseases Third edition London 1975.

Lee, G. A., SC. Leper Hospitals in Medieval Ireland, Dublin 1996.
Lenihan, Maurice, Limerick Its History and Antiquities, Cork, 1967.
Lewis, Samuel, A History and Topography of Limerick City and County, Cork 1980 pp.102 - 144.
Loudon, Irvine (ed.), Western Medicine, An Illustrated History, Oxford, 1997.
Lyons, J.B. Thrust Syphilis Down to Hell and other Rejoyceana, Dublin 1988.
Lysaght, Paddy, The House of Industry, The Old Limerick Journal No. 4, September 1980.
Notestein F. W., On Population, Three Essays Malthus, Huxley, Osborn. New York 1960.
O'Brien George, The Economic History of Ireland from the Union to the Famine, New Jersey 1972.
O'Connor, P.J. Exploring Limerick's Past: an historical geography of urban development in county and city, (Newcastle West 1987)
Ó Gráda, Cormac, Ireland A New Economic History 1780-1939, Oxford, 1994.
—. Ireland before and after the Famine, Explorations in economic history, 1800-1925, Manchester 1988.
O'Mahony, Chris, The Poor Law Comes to Limerick. The Old Limerick Journal No. 6 1980
Ó Murchadha, Ciarán, 'Limerick Union Workhouse During the Great Famine' in Old Limerick Journal Famine Edition No. 32, Winter 1995.
O'Sullivan, M. F. A history of Hospital and its environs, Tipperary 1995.
Ó Tuathaigh, Gearóid Ireland Before the Famine 1798-1848, Dublin 1991.
Orme, Nicholas and Webster, Margaret, The English Hospital: 1070-1570, London 1995.
Póirtéir, Cathal, (ed) The Great Irish Famine, Cork 1995. Famine, Fever and the Bloody Flux, Laurence M. Geary.
Porter, Dorothy Health, Civilization and the State, London 1998.
Porter, Roy (ed.), The Cambridge Illustrated History Medicine, Cambridge, 1996.
Rosenberg, C. E., Explaining Epidemics and Other Studies in the History of Medicine; Cambridge, 1992.
Smith, Dr Tony, (ed.), The British Medical Association Complete Family Health Encyclopedia, Medical Dorling Kindersley London, 1992.
Thackeray, W.M., The Irish Sketch Book, 1842, Belfast, 1985.
Tierney, Dom Mark OSB, Murroe and Boher, the history of an Irish county parish, Dublin 1966.

Tierney, Dom Mark, The Mont de Piété, and The Origins and Early Years of Barrington's Hospital in The Old Limerick Journal No. 24 1988.
Tierney, Dom Mark, The Great Famine in Murroe (1845-1849) in The Old Limerick Journal , Famine Edition No. 32, Winter 1995.
Wilson, Dr. Andrew, The Modern Physician, Vol. 1, London undated.
Wyse Jackson, Robert, The Story of Limerick; Cork 1973.